Biological Rhythms, Mood Disorders, Light Therapy, and the Pineal Gland

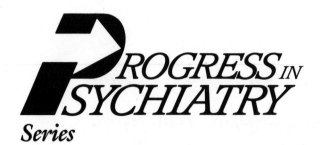

Series

David Spiegel, M.D.,
Series Editor

Biological Rhythms, Mood Disorders, Light Therapy, and the Pineal Gland

Edited by
Mohammad Shafii, M.D.
Sharon Lee Shafii, R.N., B.S.N.

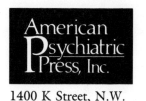

American Psychiatric Press, Inc.

1400 K Street, N.W.
Washington, DC 20005

Copyright © 1990 American Psychiatric Press, Inc.
ALL RIGHTS RESERVED
Manufactured in the United States of America
First Edition   93 92 91 90 4 3 2 1

The paper used in this publication meets the minimum requirements of the American National Standard for Information Sciences — Permanence of Paper for Printed Library Materials, ANSI Z39.48-1984.   ∞

Library of Congress Cataloging-in-Publication Data

Biological rhythms, mood disorders, light therapy, and the pineal gland / edited by Mohammad Shafii, Sharon Lee Shafii, — 1st ed.
    p.   cm. — (Progress in psychiatry.)
    Includes bibliographical references.
    ISBN 0-88048-169-2 (alk. paper)
    1. Affective disorders — Physiological aspects.
2. Pineal gland. 3. Melatonin. 4. Circadian rhythms.
5. Phototherapy. I. Shafii, Mohammad. II. Shafii, Sharon Lee. III. Series.
    [DNLM: 1. Affective Disorders — physiopathology.
2. Affective Disorders — therapy. 3. Melatonin — physiology. 4. Periodicity. 5. Phototherapy. 6. Pineal Body — physiology. 7. Pineal Body — physiopathology.
WM 171 B61486]
RC537.B497   1990
616.85'27 — dc20
DNLM/DLC
for Library of Congress   89-18447
                                               CIP

To
Husain Shafii and Naiereh Khezri
and the memory of
Arie Van Daalen and Dorothy McCabe Van Daalen,
Our Parents

Day and Man

Bright is the earth,
When thou risest in the horizon,
When thou shinest as Aton by day.
The darkness is banished,
When thou sendest forth thy rays,
The Two Lands [Egypt] are in daily festivity,
Awake and standing upon their feet,
For thou hast raised them up.
Their limbs bathed, they take their clothing;
Their arms uplifted in adoration to thy dawning.
Then in all the world, they do their work.

Day and the
Animals and Plants

All cattle rest upon their herbage,
All trees and all plants flourish,
The birds flutter in their marshes,
Their wings uplifted in adoration to thee.
All the sheep dance upon their feet,
All winged things fly,
They live when thou hast shone upon them.

Hymn to the Sun-God, Aton
Ikhnaton, Amenhotep IV of Egypt
Fourteenth century B.C.

From Breasted JH: A History of Egypt—From the Earliest Times to the Persian Conquest, 2nd Edition. New York, Charles Scribner, 1912, pp 372–373

Contents

PART II
The Pineal Gland amd Mood Disorders in Adults, Adolescents, and Children

PART III
Light Therapy and the
Pineal Gland

Contributors

Johan Beck-Friis, M.D., Ph.D.
Associate Professor in Clinical Psychiatry, Karolinska Institute, Department of Psychiatry, Stockholm, Sweden

Sarah L. Berga, M.D.
Assistant Professor of Obstetrics and Gynecology, University of Pittsburgh, School of Medicine, Pittsburgh, Pennsylvania

Kunwar P. Bhatnagar, Ph.D.
Professor of Anatomy, Department of Anatomical Sciences and Neurobiology, Health Sciences Center, University of Louisville, Louisville, Kentucky

Ann McCue Derrick, R.N., M.S.
Clinical Nurse Specialist, Child Psychiatric Services, University of Louisville School of Medicine, Louisville, Kentucky

Michael B. Foster, M.D.
Associate Professor of Pediatrics, University of Louisville, Louisville, Kentucky

J.C. Gillin, M.D.
Professor of Psychiatry, University of California, San Diego, Medical Center, San Diego, California

Richard Greenberg, Ph.D.
Professor of Community Health, School of Medicine, University of Louisville, Louisville, Kentucky

Steven P. James, M.D.
Assistant Professor of Psychiatry, University of Pennsylvania School of Medicine, Hospital of the University of Pennsylvania, Philadelphia, Pennsylvania

Mary P. Key, M.S., M.T.(ASCP)
Senior Medical Technologist, Pediatrics, University of Louisville, Louisville, Kentucky

Bengt F. Kjellman, M.D., Ph.D.
Associate Professor in Clinical Psychiatry, Karolinska Institute, Department of Psychiatry, St. Göran's Hospital, Stockholm, Sweden

Daniel F. Kripke, M.D.
Professor of Psychiatry, University of California, San Diego, Medical Center, San Diego, California

Alfred J. Lewy, M.D., Ph.D.
Professor of Psychiatry, Ophthalmology, and Pharmacology, Director, Sleep and Mood Disorders Laboratory, Director, Mass Spectrometry Laboratory, Department of Psychiatry, Oregon Health Sciences University, Portland, Oregon

Aimee Mayeda, M.D.
Assistant Professor of Psychiatry, Richard L. Roudebush Veterans Administration Medical Center, Indiana University School of Medicine, Indianapolis, Indiana

John Nurnberger, Jr., M.D., Ph.D.
Professor of Psychiatry and Neurobiology, Director, Institute of Psychiatric Research, Indiana University Medical Center, Indianapolis, Indiana

Barbara L. Parry, M.D.
Assistant Professor of Psychiatry, University of California, San Diego, Medical Center, San Diego, California

Russel J. Reiter, Ph.D.
Professor of Neuroendocrinology, Department of Cellular and Structural Biology, The University of Texas Health Science Center at San Antonio, San Antonio, Texas

Robert L. Sack, M.D.
Professor of Psychiatry, Department of Psychiatry, Oregon Health Sciences University, Portland, Oregon

Mohammad Shafii, M.D.
Professor of Psychiatry, Director, Child Psychiatry Training Program, Department of Psychiatry and Behavioral Sciences, University of Louisville, Louisville, Kentucky

Sharon Lee Shafii, R.N., B.S.N.
Editor-in-Residence, formerly Assistant Head Nurse, Adolescent Service, Neuropsychiatric Institute, University of Michigan Medical Center, Ann Arbor, Michigan

Clifford M. Singer, M.D.
Assistant Professor of Psychiatry, Department of Psychiatry, Oregon Health Sciences University, Portland, Oregon

Lennart Wetterberg, M.D., Ph.D.
Professor of Psychiatry, Karolinska Institute, Director and Chairman, Department of Psychiatry, St. Göran's Hospital, Stockholm, Sweden

Introduction to the Progress in Psychiatry Series

The *Progress in Psychiatry* Series is designed to capture in print the excitement that comes from assembling a diverse group of experts from various locations to examine in detail the newest information about a developing aspect of psychiatry. This series emerged as a collaboration between the American Psychiatric Association's (APA) Scientific Program Committee and the American Psychiatric Press, Inc. Great interest is generated by a number of the symposia presented each year at the APA Annual Meeting, and we realized that much of the information presented there, carefully assembled by people who are deeply immersed in a given area, would unfortunately not appear together in print. The symposia sessions at the Annual Meetings provide an unusual opportunity for experts who otherwise might not meet on the same platform to share their diverse viewpoints for a period of 3 hours. Some new themes are repeatedly reinforced and gain credence, while in other instances disagreements emerge, enabling the audience and now the reader to reach informed decisions about new directions in the field. The *Progress in Psychiatry* Series allows us to publish and capture some of the best of the symposia and thus provide an in-depth treatment of specific areas that might not otherwise be presented in broader review formats.

Psychiatry is by nature an interface discipline, combining the study of mind and brain, of individual and social environments, of the humane and the scientific. Therefore, progress in the field is rarely linear—it often comes from unexpected sources. Further, new developments emerge from an array of viewpoints that do not necessarily provide immediate agreement but rather expert examination of the issues. We intend to present innovative ideas and data that will enable you, the reader, to participate in this process.

We believe the *Progress in Psychiatry* Series will provide you with an opportunity to review timely new information in specific fields of interest as they are developing. We hope you find that the excitement of the presentations is captured in the written word and that this book proves to be informative and enjoyable reading.

David Spiegel, M.D.
Series Editor
Progress in Psychiatry Series

Progress in Psychiatry Series Titles

The Borderline: Current Empirical Research (#1)
Edited by Thomas H. McGlashan, M.D.

**Premenstrual Syndrome: Current Findings and Future
Directions (#2)**
Edited by Howard J. Osofsky, M.D., Ph.D., and Susan J.
Blumenthal, M.D.

Treatment of Affective Disorders in the Elderly (#3)
Edited by Charles A. Shamoian, M.D.

Post-Traumatic Stress Disorder in Children (#4)
Edited by Spencer Eth, M.D., and Robert S. Pynoos, M.D., M.P.H.

The Psychiatric Implications of Menstruation (#5)
Edited by Judith H. Gold, M.D., F.R.C.P. (C)

Can Schizophrenia Be Localized in the Brain? (#6)
Edited by Nancy C. Andreasen, M.D., Ph.D.

Medical Mimics of Psychiatric Disorders (#7)
Edited by Irl Extein, M.D., and Mark S. Gold, M.D.

Biopsychosocial Aspects of Bereavement (#8)
Edited by Sidney Zisook, M.D.

Psychiatric Pharmacosciences of Children and Adolescents (#9)
Edited by Charles Popper, M.D.

Psychobiology of Bulimia (#10)
Edited by James I. Hudson, M.D., and Harrison G. Pope, Jr., M.D.

Cerebral Hemisphere Function in Depression (#11)
Edited by Marcel Kinsbourne, M.D.

Eating Behavior in Eating Disorders (#12)
Edited by B. Timothy Walsh, M.D.

**Tardive Dyskinesia: Biological Mechanisms and Clinical
Aspects (#13)**
Edited by Marion E. Wolf, M.D., and Aron D. Mosnaim, Ph.D.

Current Approaches to the Prediction of Violence (#14)
Edited by David A. Brizer, M.D., and Martha L. Crowner, M.D.

Treatment of Tricyclic-Resistant Depression (#15)
Edited by Irl L. Extein, M.D.

Depressive Disorders and Immunity (#16)
Edited by Andrew H. Miller, M.D.

Introduction

Humans throughout the millennium have been fascinated and mystified by the effect of the sun, moon, and stars on their daily lives. The day-night cycle and seasonal changes have been the source of adoration, religious beliefs, and "scientific" exploration since time began.

In recent years, for the first time in the history of science, we are moving from anecdotal observations to replicable, scientifically based investigations of the relationship between living organisms and the light-dark cycle (circadian rhythm) and seasonal changes (circannual), now referred to as chronobiology—the study of biological rhythms.

With advances in molecular and cellular biology, neuroendocrinology, neurobiology, and psychoneuroimmunology, we are beginning to bridge the chasm between the mind-body duality that has plagued Western sciences for more than 300 years. According to Hall (1989), "Only with the convergence of molecular biology, immunology, and neuroscience have scientists begun to span the huge gap between emotions, mental processes and molecules" (p. 66).

The use of psychopharmacological agents in psychiatry has opened new vistas to researchers and clinicians regarding the role of neurotransmitters, not only in the central nervous system, but throughout the whole organism. Increased emphasis on phenomenologically oriented diagnostic criteria based on clinical observations and use of statistical methods for inclusion or exclusion of specific criteria has significantly enhanced the research clinician's capability for scientific validation.

Many believe we are on the threshold of a profound revolution in the fields of the neurosciences, psychiatry, and human behavior. Development of new methodology such as radioimmunoassay and gas chromatography–mass spectrometry is helping researchers and clinicians measure minute amounts of hormones and other chemical products in the central nervous system, endocrine system, and body fluids, which until recently was impossible.

Compared with other endocrine glands such as the pituitary, thyroid, and adrenal glands, study of the pineal gland and its function in health and disorder has been neglected. With the pioneering work of Lerner, Axelrod, Wurtman, Vaughan, Waldhauser, Arendt, Reiter, Wetterberg, Lewy, Rosenthal, Kripke, Wehr, and others, the pineal gland and its function in psychiatric disorders such as depressive disorders, bipolar disorders, premenstrual syndrome, and sleep disorders have become the focus of scientific and clinical investigation. We now know that the pineal gland, in addition to being an independent pacesetter and timekeeper, is via the suprachiasmatic nucleus of the hypothalamus a photosensitive organ which translates environmental messages of the light-dark cycle and seasonal changes into hormonal messages sent throughout the living organism.

Biological Rhythms, Mood Disorders, Light Therapy, and the Pineal Gland brings to psychiatric clinicians, adult, child, and adolescent psychiatric residents, medical students, and other health professionals the progress made in the study of the pineal gland and its relationship to mood disorders, including major depressive disorders, winter depression, bipolar disorders, premenstrual syndrome, and sleep disorders. Recent developments in the use of bright light in the treatment of these disorders are discussed.

The book is divided into three parts. In Part I, "Comparative Morphology and Physiology of the Pineal Gland," the general features of the pineal gland from lampreys to mammals are briefly reviewed. The human pineal gland and its development throughout the life cycle, gross anatomy, and cellular structure are succinctly but comprehensively examined. The physiology of the pineal gland including pineal rhythmicity and the neuroendocrine and behavioral effects of the pineal hormone melatonin are explored. Part I lays the foundation for the subsequent chapters.

In Part II, "The Pineal Gland and Mood Disorders in Adults, Adolescents, and Children," recent research in correlating the levels of serum and/or urinary melatonin with mood disorders, particularly major depressive disorders and bipolar disorders, and primary depression in children and adolescents is reviewed and discussed. Although the exploration of the relationship between the pineal gland and mood disorders is in an early stage, exciting possibilities exist for future discovery in this area.

In Part III, "Light Therapy and the Pineal Gland," we see the integration of research findings on the pineal gland and biological rhythms with clinical practice in the form of bright-light therapy in the treatment of winter depression, premenstrual syndrome, and sleep disorders.

The editing of this book began while we were on sabbatical and residing during the winter months of 1989 in Nice, Côte d'Azur, France, the city of sun and flowers as immortalized by Marc Chagall in his paintings. During this sabbatical, we also had an opportunity to visit the Lascaux II cave paintings in the valley of the Vézères River close to Périgueux in southwestern France. These cave paintings made by our ancestors between 20,000 and 15,000 years ago, perhaps in anticipation of the transmigration of animals due to seasonal changes during the Ice Age, inspired us beyond our imagination.

We are grateful to Carol Nadelson, M.D., Editor-in-Chief, and David Spiegel, M.D., Editor of the *Progress in Psychiatry* Series, of the American Psychiatric Press, Inc., for their receptivity and support for the publication of this book. We are also thankful to Amy Willard, Program and Research Assistant, for her attention to detail, for cross-checking the accuracy of references, and for carefully and speedily typing the manuscript.

Mohammad and Sharon Shafii

REFERENCE
Hall SS: A molecular code links emotions, mind and health. Smithsonian 20:62–71, 1989

PART I

Comparative Morphology and Physiology of the Pineal Gland

Chapter 1

Comparative Morphology of the Pineal Gland

Kunwar P. Bhatnagar, Ph.D.

Chapter 1

Comparative Morphology of the Pineal Gland

Our knowledge of the structure and function of the human pineal gland is far from being complete, even though numerous reports, books, symposia proceedings, well-compiled treatises (e.g., Kitay and Altschule 1954; Reiter 1984; Vollrath 1981), research review series, and a specialty journal have brought this enigmatic organ to the forefront of science. Most of the information available on the human pineal is primarily pathological in nature. This review provides a summary understanding of the pineal organ in the entire vertebrate series, focusing principally on what is known about the human pineal and what more remains to be known.

Among vertebrates, the pineal gland makes its first appearance in lampreys and, with certain exceptions (Ralph 1984; Vollrath 1981) that may be doubtful, is found in all species. Schematized drawings of the pineal region of representative vertebrates (Figure 1-1) and a comparison of the general features of the pineal organ (Table 1-1) are provided for an overview highlighting the evolutionary trends of the pineal from lampreys to mammals. Vollrath (1981) offers an excellent review and summary.

THE MAMMALIAN PINEAL GLAND

A pineal gland is present in all mammalian species beginning with the two monotremes, the marsupials (some of which reportedly lack a pineal), and the rest of the eutherian orders (Kenny and Scheelings

I am grateful to Dr. Subhash C. Sharma, Sparrow Hospital, Lansing, Michigan; to David Krause, M.D., for the CT scans in Figure 1-6; and to Dr. Kenneth C. Leskawa for help in organizing Table 1-3. Bob Knaster photographed the human half-brain preparation. Human pineal material for this study was obtained from cadavers through the courtesy of Dr. S.A. Larsen and Mr. William Duvall. The typescript was meticulously prepared by Susan Hodge.

Table 1-1. General features of vertebrate pineal gland[a]

	Lampreys	Fish	Amphibians	Reptiles	Birds	Mammals
Gross anatomy	Epiphyseal complex consisting of pineal organ proper and				Epiphysis cerebri	
	Parapineal organ; adult *Myxine* lacks pineal	Parapineal organ	Extracranial frontal organ; additional pineal	Parietal or the third eye in lacertilians	Accessory pineal tissue	
Pineal organ pointing	Anteriad	Anteriad	Anteriad	Vertical and anteriad	Mostly vertical	Posteriad
Hollow vs. solid	Hollow	Hollow to compact	Hollow to compact	Hollow	Saccular	Solid
Position in relation to skull	Close to skull	Close to skull	Deeper to skull	Deep to the skull roof	Deep to the skull roof	Superficial to deeply situated under cover of cerebral hemispheres. Exception is certain bats.[b]

Structural organization	Photoreceptor cells, supporting cells, and intrapineal nerve cells poor or lacking in Nissl substance; "pineal window"			Photoreceptor cells; supporting cells	Photoreceptor cells; supporting cells; lymphoid tissue	Pinealocytes; glial cells; intrapineal neurons in association with blood vessels.[b] Acervuli in some species.
Afferent fibers	Predominate	Predominate; pineal tract	Predominate; pineal tract	Pineal tract	Reduced	Lacking
Efferent fibers	?	Doubtful	?	Regularly seen	Densely innervate	Predominate
Function	Photosensory; secretory; color change	Photosensory; secretory; color change	Photosensory; secretory	Photosensory; secretory	Light sensitive; secretory	Light sensitive; secretory
Secretory or synthesized product	Melatonin	Melatonin	Melatonin	Melatonin	Melatonin	Melatonin

[a]Vollrath 1981. [b]Bhatnagar 1988; Bhatnagar et al. 1986, in press.

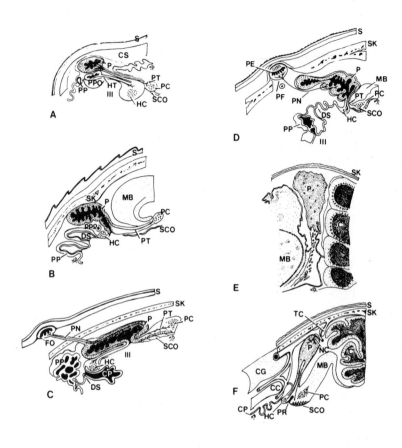

Figure 1-1.   Schematic representation of sagittal sections through pineal region of lamprey (*A*); teleost fish (*B*); frog (*C*); lizard (*D*); bird, a cormorant (*E*); and rat (*F*) to show pineal, parapineal, and other related components as they appear in phylogeny. *A–D* and *F* are modified from Wurtman et al. (1968) and *E* is based on Quay (1965). C, cerebellum; CC, corpus callosum; CG, cingulate gyrus; CP, choroid plexus; CS, cartilaginous skull; DS, dorsal sac; FO, frontal (parapineal) organ; HC, habenular commissure; HT, habenular tract; MB, midbrain; NC, nervi conarii; P, pineal organ; PC, posterior commissure; PE, parietal eye; PF, parietal foramen; PN, pineal nerve; PP, paraphysis; PPO, parapineal organ; PR, pineal recess; PT, pineal tract; S, skin; SCO, subcommissural organ; SK, skull; TC, tentorium cerebelli; III, third ventricle.

1979; Vollrath 1981). A brief description of the general features of the pineal gland can be found in Table 1-1. Until recently, information on the pineal gland of bats was sporadic and even erroneous. In our laboratory, comparative studies on a large number of species of bats have established the highly variable and hitherto undescribed features of the pineal morphology of bats (Bhatnagar 1988; Bhatnagar et al. 1985–1986, 1986, in press; Chang et al. 1987). Space restrictions limit further discussion even of general features of the mammalian pineal gland. Therefore, the rest of this review will primarily be devoted to the human pineal gland.

ABSENCE OF THE PINEAL GLAND

The pineal gland is reportedly lacking in some species, such as crocodilians, anteaters, sloths, armadillos, the marsupial *Petaurus* (Vollrath 1979), and some bats (Bhatnagar et al. 1986). Several factors may have led to such assumptions. The pineal gland is diffuse in a few species (such as in *Dasypus, Loxodonta,* and *Hyrax* [Vollrath 1979]) and therefore difficult to identify. Also, often not enough specimens of a species are examined systematically, resulting in erroneous conclusions. Furthermore, if indeed the pineal gland is lacking in a species, a detailed investigation of the embryonic development of the brain should be mandatory in establishing whether there ever was a pineal anlage and, if so, at what stage during development it was lost. In these extreme cases, the investigator needs to explore the relations of the habenular and posterior commissures, which are related to the pineal stalk in most species.

THE HUMAN PINEAL GLAND

Development

The pineal gland, which is one of the circumventricular organs, arises as an evagination of the roof of the third ventricle at the beginning of the second month of gestation (33rd postovulatory day) (Hülsemann 1971; O'Rahilly 1968). Through cell proliferation and growth of the ependyma, the pineal anlage, which consists of two to three separate lobes, fuses to form a solid mass into which vascular connective tissue grows, thus giving the pineal parenchyma a lobular appearance. During further development, the pineal gland changes its axis from vertical to horizontal. The pineal gland receives its innervation prenatally.

Evolutionary considerations reveal the pineal gland to be an integral part of the photoneuroendocrine system in all classes of vertebrates, from lampreys to mammals, with major differences (Collin and

Oksche 1981; Scharrer 1964). The pineal gland, closely related to and an integral part of the optic pathway, is established by its presence as a discreet organ in all vertebrates beginning with lampreys who are endowed with visual systems. Even in invertebrate orders Arthropoda and Mollusca, visual elements are present in their well-defined optic systems. Optic lobes of cockroaches are the sites of circadian pacemakers (Edmunds 1988; Page 1982). Takahashi and Menaker (1984) have demonstrated the capacities for circadian oscillation and photoreception throughout the chicken pineal gland, and even small pieces of the pineal gland produced circadian oscillation. It would be interesting to know if pineal secretory products have a common basis in all animals, both invertebrates and vertebrates, in possession of visual systems.

Neonatal Human Pineal Gland

Pineal glands of 16 infants ranging from 38 weeks gestation to 3 years of age were examined by Min et al. (1987), who observed two types of cells. Type I cells, predominant at birth and frequently pigmented, were positive for S-100 protein and negative for neuron-specific enolase. The type II cells were strongly positive for neuron-specific enolase and negative for melanin and S-100 protein. At 1 year postnatally, few S-100 protein–positive cells remained, with the bulk formed by type II cells, the pinealocytes. These observations led the authors to conclude that the human pineal gland undergoes a significant morphologic transformation during early childhood.

A steady decline of serum melatonin was observed by Gupta (1985) in a series of hospitalized but endocrinologically healthy patients ranging from preschool to sexually mature ages. Serum melatonin night values showed an increment from the 3rd month postnatally through preschool age. These observations are suggestive of a relationship between the pineal gland (and other melatonin producing-synthesizing organs such as retina) and the developmental process in general—not specifically limited to sexual development.

Bartsch and Bartsch (1985) observed rhythmic melatonin production by the end of the 3rd week of postnatal life, in contrast to Gupta (1985), who reported an absence of circadian rhythm in the 1st month of life. Also, Gupta noticed night peaking of melatonin during the 2nd and 3rd month of life, although circadian rhythm was not fully established.

Bartsch and Bartsch (1985) reported that maternal melatonin crosses the placenta. After birth, maternal melatonin reaches the neonate through the milk. Whether lactating women have been assayed for their milk melatonin levels is unknown to me. Studies of milk melatonin levels at different stages of lactation should help in understanding pineal function.

Gross Structure

The human pineal (epiphysis cerebri) is a major component of the epithalamus along with the habenular trigones, the striae medullares thalami, and the epithelial roof of the third ventricle. It is a small, flattened, pinecone-shaped structure lying horizontally in the superior subarachnoid cistern in the space between the splenium of the corpus callosum and the superior colliculi (Figure 1-2, Table 1-2). Its relations are the thalamic pulvinar laterally, cerebellum posteriorly, the habenular trigone anteriorly, and the posterior commissure and superior colliculi inferiorly (Figure 1-2). The splenium of the corpus callosum abuts the pineal superiorly. Its base is hollow and pedunculated, by which it is attached to the roof of the third ventricle. The latter extends into the stalk as the pineal recess of the third ventricle. Additionally, a suprapineal recess of the third ventricle overlies the pineal. Often it is stated that the pineal gland is bathed in the cerebrospinal fluid (CSF). However, the pineal is no more in contact with the CSF than any other brain surface, because the gland is encapsulated within a pial sheath which is bathed by CSF in the subarachnoid space.

The pineal is spheroid in the newborn (Sparks and Hunsaker 1988). It reaches adult size around the 4th year of life (Gudernatsch 1953). According to Tapp (1986), no significant histological or structural changes occur in the pineal from childhood to old age other than those associated with aging in general. The cytoglandular architecture is highly variable from one gland to the other as well as within the gland itself (Tapp 1979); such is the case with the weight and dimensions of the pineal also. Some authors, such as Gudernatsch (1953), have commented on the extremely high variability of the pineal gland and compared it with other organs that have peaked on the phylogenetic scale and that are now destined for fading out. I do not hold these views.

The pineal comprises primarily clusters of parenchymal cells—the pinealocytes—enclosed within bands of connective tissue of variable thickness (Figure 1-3). Glial cells, which are mainly fibrous astrocytes, are present in much fewer numbers. Other cells that are infrequently seen include lymphocytes, oligodendrocytes associated with central commissural fibers, Schwann cells associated with sympathetic innervation to the pineal, mast cells, macrophages, pigment cells, connective tissue elements, and occasional neurons. Several calibers of blood vessels are profusely distributed. Based on animal studies, even in-

Table 1-2. Biological data on human pineal gland

Shape	Pinecone-shaped	Vollrath 1979
Pineal type	A	
Dimensions[a]		
Height, maximum width	8.8 mm, 5.2 mm	Bhatnagar, this study
Weight[b]	138.6 mg	Legait and Legait 1977
	109.25 mg	Bhatnagar, this study
Volume	46.12 mm^3	Legait et al. 1976a, 1976b
Ratio of pineal weight to brain weight during ages 41–50	1:8240	Von Eyl and Gusek 1975
First appearance in embryo	33rd postovulatory day (6–8 mm crown-rump length)	O'Rahilly 1968
Substances identified in pineal body		
Low-molecular-mass endothelial cell–stimulating angiogenic factor	5.43 ± 1.92 μg (n = 3 subjects) collagen degraded per hour per mg protein in 20,000 g supernatant	Taylor et al. 1988
Melatonin levels[c] by radioimmunoassay (daytime/nighttime)	0–20/46 ± 4.8 pg/ml	Waldhauser et al. 1984a, 1984b, 1987; Waldhauser and Gisinger 1986; also see Wetterberg 1981

RNA content		
Total pineal	15.89 µg/mg dry weight	Landolt et al. 1966
Individual pinealocyte	11.00 pg	
DNA content		
Total pineal	10.13 µg/mg dry weight	Landolt et al. 1966
Ganglioside *N*-acetylneuraminic acid (NeuNAc)	0.042% of dry weight	Landolt et al. 1966
Cerebrosides	7.2 pg/cell, 1.1% dry weight	Landolt and Hess 1966
Cholesterol	3.4 mg/g fresh tissue	Czarnocki et al. 1969
Lipid content	Variable: 2.9%	Basinka et al. 1969
	9.2%	Czarnocki et al. 1969
Proteolipid protein	1.57% dry weight or 10.2 pg/cell	Landolt and Hess 1966
Human neurophysin I		Gauquelin et al. 1982
Males	47 ng/gland	
Females	24 ng/gland	
Human neurophysin II		Gauquelin et al. 1982
Males	7 ng/gland	
Females	15 ng/gland	

[a] Often, pineal dimensions are given for length, width, and height. Because the usual shape of a pineal gland is conical, the approximate dimensions are only two — height and base or maximum width. All dimensions are extremely variable so much so that there could hardly be a true average dimension.

[b] Pineal weight in humans is highly variable and subject to the degree of calcification (Tapp and Huxley 1972). It is much lower after decalcification.

[c] Highly variable levels of melatonin have been reported by various workers (see Waldhauser et al. 1984a, 1984b). The values quoted here are just one set of data from a laboratory active in research on melatonin. Melatonin production has been reported to decline with age (Sack et al. 1986).

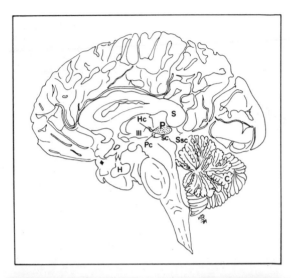

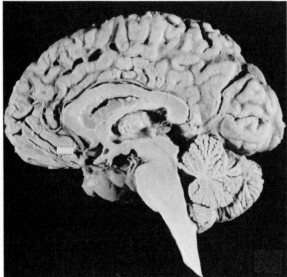

Figure 1-2. Medial surface of the right hemisphere of the human brain. C, cerebellum; H, hypophysis; Hc, habenular commissure; P, pineal gland, Pc, posterior commissure; S, splenium of the corpus callosum; SC, superior colliculus; Ssc, superior subarachnoid cistern; III, third ventricle. Scale in bottom half shows 1-mm divisions.

trapineal expression of striated muscle can be expected (Quay 1959). Indeed, striated muscle has been reported in the human pineal (see Vollrath 1981).

Calcareous concretions (sand granules, brain sand, corpora arenacea, or acervuli) are mulberry-shaped bodies within the pineal and show concentric growth zones in sections (Figure 1-4). These concretions are not universally present in the pineals of all vertebrates, and their significance is poorly understood. The concretions consist of mineral deposits such as phosphates of calcium, magnesium, and ammonium and calcium carbonate. In the Mongolian gerbil, the first calcification sites have been found in the cytoplasmic matrix, vacuoles, mitochondria, and the endoplasmic reticulum (Krstić 1986). These loci develop into a concretion by addition of hydroxyapatite crystals, causing the cell finally to die. The acervuli reach the extracellular space. Much remains to be learned about the pineal concretions because they are not found in many species, for example in most bats (Bhatnagar et al. 1986).

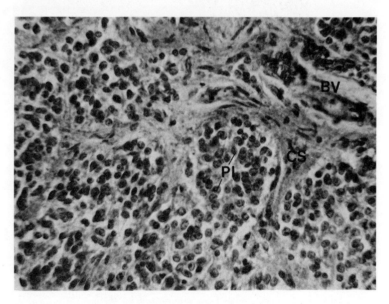

Figure 1-3.   Light micrograph of section through human pineal gland. Note connective tissue septa (CS), with blood vessels (BV), surrounding clusters of pinealocytes (PI). 8 μm; hematoxylin and eosin; x320.

Branches of the posterior cerebral arteries, the posterolateral central arteries, provide the arterial blood to the pineal (Ganti et al. 1986, Figure 9D; Walls 1964, p. 882), whereas the enormous venous return is into the great cerebral vein of Galen. The profuse venous pattern is suggestive of a functional role in the pineal for facilitating the distribution of synthesized materials (Table 1-3), such as serotonin, melatonin, and the enzyme hydroxyindole-0-methyltransferase (HIOMT), which synthesizes melatonin from serotonin (see Chapter 2). Elegant studies by Wiechman et al. (1985) on the human and bovine pineal gland and retina have localized the enzyme HIOMT in both pinealocytes and photoreceptors. Lymphatics are not present in the pineal (Diehl 1978).

Pinealocytes

Pinealocytes are large parenchymal cells with a prominent nucleus and a nucleolus (Figure 1-5). Generally, they exhibit several cytoplasmic

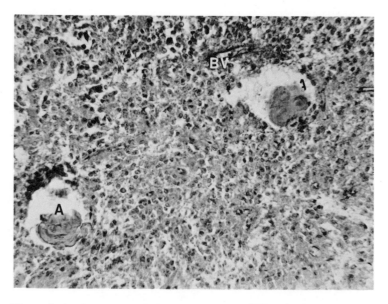

Figure 1-4. Low-power light micrograph of section through human pineal. Two acervuli (A) show their concentrically layered structure. Note that these corpora arenacea are lying free in spaces devoid of any cellular matter. BV, blood vessel. 8 μm; Masson trichrome; x200.

Table 1-3. Partial list of substances identified within mammalian pineal gland (see Vollrath 1981; Quay 1981)

INORGANIC SALTS
  Calcium (Ca^{2+})
  Cobalt
  Copper
  Iron
  Manganese
  Phosphorus
  Rubidium
  Selenium
  Strontium
  Sulfur
  Zinc
  Magnesium (Mg^{2+})
  Potassium (K^+)
  Sodium (Na^+)

PIGMENTS
  Melanin
  Lipofuscin
  Hemosiderin

PEPTIDES AND PROTEINS
  Adrenocorticotropic hormone
    (ACTH)
  Angiotensin I and II
  Arginine vasopressin
  Arginine vasotocin
  Estradiol
  Gonadotropin-inhibiting
    substance
  Lipotropins
  Luteinizing hormone–releasing
    hormone (LHRH)
  α-Melanocyte-stimulating
    hormone (MSH)

Neurophysin I and II (human)
Oxytocin
Progesterone
Somatostatin
Thyrotropin-releasing hormone
  (TRH)
Vasoactive intestinal peptide
  (VIP)
Vasotocin
Endothelial cell–stimulating
  angiogenic factor (ESAF)[a]

ENZYMES
  Oxidoreductases
  Alcohol dehydrogenase
  Lactate dehydrogenase
  β-Hydroxybutyrate
    dehydrogenase
  Malate dehydrogenase
  6-Phosphogluconic
    dehydrogenase
  Glucose-6-phosphate
    dehydrogenase
  Steroid dehydrogenase
  α-Glycerophosphate
    dehydrogenase
  Glyceraldehyde phosphate
    dehydrogenase
  Succinate dehydrogenase
  Glutamate dehydrogenase
  Monoamine oxidase
  NADPH diaphorase
  Cytochrome oxidase
  Peroxidase

Table 1-3. Partial list of substances identified within mammalian pineal gland (continued)

Transferases
Hydroxyindole-*O*-methyltransferase (HIOMT)
N-acetyltransferase
Phosphorylase

Hydrolases
Nonspecific esterases
Lipase
Acetylcholinesterase
Nonspecific cholinesterase
Alkaline phosphatase
Acid phosphatase
5'-Nucleotidase
Glucose-6-phosphatase
Arylsulfatase
β-Glucuronidase
Leucine aminopeptidase
Adenosine triphosphatase (ATPase)
Nucleosidediphosphatase
Thiamine pyrophosphatase

Lyases
Aldolase
Carbonic anhydrase
Adenylyl cyclase
5-Hydroxytryptophan decarboxylase

IMMUNOREACTIVE PROTEINS
Alpha-transducin
S-100 protein
Glial fibrillary acidic (GFA) protein
Intermediate-filament–associated protein
48 kD protein
Anti-LHRH
Anti-TRH
Interstitial retinol-binding protein
Cellular retinal-binding protein
Immunoreactive opsin
Rhodopsin kinase

NUCLEIC ACIDS
DNA
RNA

COMPLEX CARBOHYDRATES
Glycogen
Glycoproteins
Proteoglycan (mucopolysaccharides)
Cerebrosides
Gangliosides

OTHER LIPIDS
Cholesterol
Phospholipids
Sphingomyelin
Triglycerides
Fatty acids

Table 1-3. Partial list of substances identified within mammalian pineal gland (continued)

FREE AMINO ACIDS	HORMONE RECEPTORS FOR
Aliphatic amino acids	Estradiol[b]
Arginine	Progesterone[b]
Cystathionine	Prostaglandins[b]
Glycine	Glucocorticoids[c]
Histidine	
Lysine	
Methionine	OTHER SUBSTANCES
S-Adenosyl methionine	Ascorbic acid
Taurine	Inositol
Tryptophan	Cyclic nucleotides (cAMP, cGMP)
Amino acid derivative	Adenosine
	Prostaglandins[d]
NEUROTRANSMITTER AND SECRETORY PRODUCTS	Carbolines
Serotonin	Amyloid deposits
Melatonin	Hydroxyapatite
Dopamine	Calcareous concretions (acervuli)
Histamine	
Epinephrine	OTHER BLOOD-BORNE ELEMENTS
Norepinephrine	
γ-Aminobutyric acid (GABA)	FICTITIOUS PRODUCTS
Glutamate	Volvolon[e]
Acetylcholine	

[a]Taylor et al. 1988. [b]Cardinali et al. 1982. [c]Demisch et al. 1987. [d]Cardinali and Ritta 1983. [e]This substance is fictitious. Obviously, its creation was intended to provide amusement to jaded scientists (Iversen 1982). Another article that belongs to this category is by Bayliss et al. (1985; personal communication).

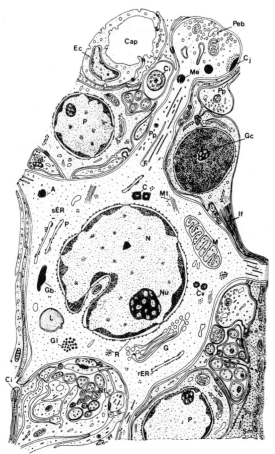

Figure 1-5. Schematic and idealized ultrastructural representation of human pinealocytes (P) and adjacent interstitial components based primarily on descriptions by Møller (1974, 1976) and Hülsemann (1971). A, acervuli (early stage); C, centrioles; Cap, capillary; Ci, cilium; Cj, "intermediate-type" cell junction; Cv, coated vesicles; Ec, endothelial cell; F, filaments; G, Golgi complex; Gb, granular body; Gc, glial cell; Gl, glycogen; If, intermediate filaments; L, lysosome; M, mitochondria; Me, melanin granules; Mt, microtubules; N, nucleus; Nf, nerve fibers; Nu, nucleolus; P, pinealocyte; Peb, pinealocyte end bulb; Pp, pinealocyte process; R, ribosomes; rER, sER, rough and smooth endoplasmic reticulum; Sm, striated muscle fibers in cross section.

processes that terminate in club-shaped endings close to or within the numerous perivascular spaces (Karasek 1987). Whether all pinealocytes are multipolar remains an open question. A recent report characterizing the membrane currents in dissociated adult rat pineal cells (*pinealocytes*, implication mine) portrayed the pineal cell in a scanning electron micrograph as having surface membrane–coated blebs and occasional microvilli. Only 1 of 70 such cells showed a projection contacting a neighboring pineal cell (Aguayo and Weight 1988). This so-called pineal cell, in my opinion, appears similar to one of the formed elements of the blood, most likely a lymphocyte, and not a pineal cell.

The cytoplasmic organelles are not randomly distributed, but form clusters in the so-called anuclear region (Møller 1974, 1976). This clustering of organelles is not unusual and can even be expected because most of the space is taken by the huge nuclei, which are extensively folded. Cytoplasmic organelles include multilamellated Golgi complex producing smooth and coated vesicles, moderate amounts of rough endoplasmic reticulum generally restricted to the terminal pinealocytic endings, microtubules and neurofilaments, polyribosomes, glycogen deposits, vacuoles, occasionally present lipid droplets and lysosomes, centrioles, and cilia (Vollrath 1984). Dense-core vesicles are fewer in number. Synaptic ribbons or vesicle-crowned rodlets are present conspicuously. These cytoplasmic organelles (Figure 1-5) are said to be involved in interpinealocytic communication or otherwise participate in controlling the number of β-adrenergic receptors on the pinealocyte membrane (King and Dougherty 1982).

Glial Cells

Also known as fibrous astrocytes or interstitial cells, glial cells are the second and the only other major component of the human pineal. The following account is based on work by Papasozomenos (1983, 1986). The differentiation of pinealocytes and astrocytes becomes apparent around the 32nd week of gestation, where astrocytic development seems to lag behind that of the pinealocytes. The process of differentiation in the pineal gland is completed around the 9th month postnatally. The pineal astrocytes are readily identifiable at this time, comprising a smaller and darker nuclei as compared with the pinealocytes, which have larger and lighter nuclei. Even though impregnation techniques such as those of gold chloride sublimate or silver carbonate have been applied to the study of astrocytes, these techniques, lacking the specificity of metallic impregnation, leave doubts regarding the nature of the impregnated cells. The use of glial fibrillary acidic (GFA) protein staining technique is recognized as an ideal and specific marker for glial filaments in astrocytes (Bignami et al. 1980; Eng and DeArmond 1982). A 48 kilodalton intermediate-filament–associated protein that is different than the GFA protein in mouse brain astrocytes is involved in providing more tensile strength to the cytoplasm (Abd-El-Basset et al. 1988).

Fibrous astrocytes abundant in the human pineal show ramifying processes that enclose groups of pinealocytes (Hülsemann 1967). Some glial fibers in animals arise from the surrounding extrapineal structures reaching the pineal gland where they form astrocytic end feet terminating in close proximity to the perivascular spaces (Vollrath 1981). Wartenberg (1968) has reported the presence of intermediate filaments in the cat astrocytic processes. Their presence in the pinealocytes has been established in the vampire bat (Bhatnagar 1988). Compared with the pinealocytes, the pineal astrocytes exhibit larger amounts of condensed chromatin, less infolded nuclei, and larger amounts of rough endoplasmic reticulum and lysosomes. Mitochondria are smaller and electron dense. Much remains to be discovered with regard to their detailed ultrastructure. As for other glia, a supportive role for pineal astrocytes is postulated, and the possibilities for an active metabolic role for them are also suggested (Papasozomenos 1983).

Innervation

There is as much variability and confusion of interpretation concerning innervation of the pineal gland as there is in the knowledge about pineal function. Both pinealofugal and pinealopetal innervation have been described (Korf et al. 1986). The best-documented (but with many questions still remaining) principal innervation of the pineal is through the general visceral efferent sympathetic system, which originates as a postganglionic pathway in the superior cervical sympathetic ganglia reaching the pineal through the yet to be fully understood nervi conarii. Within the pineal, these unmyelinated fibers are seen in bundles in the connective tissue and the perivascular spaces. These nerve bundles consist of fibers highly variable in diameter. Occasionally, single-nerve fibers in the intercellular space are also encountered between the parenchymal elements, generally the pinealocytes. Despite the nerve-fiber bundles that are seen in large numbers, synaptic formations are surprisingly rare. Axosomatic and axoaxonal synapses have been reported in monkeys (Ichimura et al. 1986), in vampire bats (Bhatnagar 1988), and in the "pineal nerve" of the human fetus (Møller 1978).

Parasympathetic innervation to the pineal gland has also been claimed (Vollrath 1981). However, such innervation remains questionable as does the pinealopetal innervation, which may, at the very best, involve aberrant nerve cells displaced from habenular nuclei and their central processes. The habenular and posterior commissures are intimately related to the pineal base, but they may not traverse through the gland itself in the same manner as they do in some animals (for example, in the mouse-tailed bat [Bhatnagar et al. 1985–1986] and other bats [Bhatnagar et al. 1986]). Extension of habenular fibers through the proximal parts of the pineal in the human fetus was reported by Hülsemann (1971). Intrapineal nerve cell bodies and ganglionic structures have been described and are variously interpreted (Vollrath 1981). However, because these occur in juxtaposition with the blood vessels (Bhatnagar 1988; Bhatnagar et al. 1986, in press), they are considered to be autonomic in nature and to have a role in the control of blood flow through the pineal.

Pineal Calcification

Acervuli are found in the cellular areas as well as in the pineal connective tissue (Tapp 1979). Cysts are commonly seen in the pineal gland (Tapp 1979). Pineal calcification exists to the extent of 3% in the first 12 months postnatally, rising to 7.1% at 10 years of age and up to 33% at 18 years of age, as reported by Helmke and Winkler (1986). They point out that the presence of pineal calcification even very early in infancy might be physiological.

A computed tomographic (CT) investigation of pineal calcification in 77 patients (of 725 examined) from 6.5 to 20 years of age by Zimmerman and Bilaniuk (1982) suggests a possible relationship between calcification and the hormonal role of the pineal in regulating sexual development. Pineal calcification incidence is highly variable for different populations of the world, being lower in American blacks (9.7%), higher for Indians (19–24%), and extremely high in Ugandans (68%) in pineals removed at autopsy (Michotte et al. 1977; Zimmerman and Bilaniuk 1982). The weight of pineal calcification in women decreases after menopause, beginning at age 60 (Tapp and Huxley 1972).

Commentz et al. (1985) determined the long-term effects of cranial irradiation on pineal function by measuring melatonin levels and concluded that cranial irradiation and chemotherapy do not effect the pineal secretory pattern of melatonin circadian rhythm.

Pineal Tumors

The most common pineal tumor is the nonparenchymal germinoma, which forms about 75% of all pineal tumors (Clarke 1988; Kilgore et al. 1986; Tapp 1979; Trentini et al. 1986).

Pineal-region tumors (Figure 1-6) present manifestations of increased intracranial pressure, such as Parinaud's syndrome, hydrocephalus, and a mass in the posterior third ventricle region. Ventricular shunting, craniotomy, and subtotal resection followed by postoperative irradiation (between 30 and 55 Gy) often are the treatments of choice, with a 10-year survival rate in 67% of patients (Amendola et al. 1984). Vertebral angiography successfully demonstrates that the tumor mass is fed by the hypertrophied posterior cerebral and choroidal arteries (Ganti et al. 1986). Germinomas respond best to radiation therapy (Futrell et al. 1981).

The pineal gland is implicated in breast cancer (Cohen et al. 1978). Lehrer et al. (1985) reported an abnormally diminished sense of smell in women with estrogen-receptor–positive breast cancer, thus corroborating the relation between the pineal gland and the sense of smell.

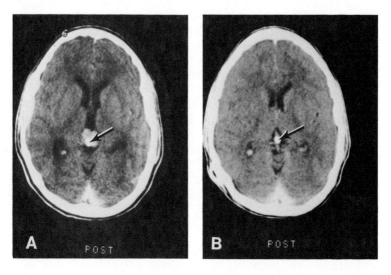

Figure 1-6.   Pineal-region tumor in 15-year-old boy. Horizontal computed tomographic scan shows pineal-region lesion (*A*) with no obstructive changes other than widened third ventricle. Two months later, postradiation (5000 rads) scan (*B*) shows regression of tumor. Calcified pineal gland (*arrow*) is prominently seen. Courtesy of David Krause, M.D., and Subhash Sharma, Ph.D., Sparrow Hospital, Lansing, Michigan.

Pineal-Region Lesions

Space-occupying tumorous, cystic, or vascular lesions of the pineal region are not uncommon, accounting for 5% of intracranial tumors in children (Hoffman 1984). Until recently, these were inoperable, but, with the advent of CT and magnetic resonance imaging and advances in anesthesiology and intensive care, such tumors are now safely surgically treated with good results after infratentorial-supracerebellar, left transventricular, and right parietal-transcallosal approaches for lesions identified as pineoblastoma, pineolocytoma, glious cyst, and other lesions (Borit and Schmidek 1984; Vorkapic and Pendl 1987).

High serum melatonin levels have been implicated as a pineal tumor marker (Miles et al. 1985); however, Vorkapic and Pendl (1987) were unable to establish high levels of melatonin in several patients with pineal tumors (Bruckner et al. 1986).

Age-Related Changes in Pineal Structure

Estimation of the nuclear-to-cytoplasmic material ratio in pinealocytes in patients 30–40 years of age and those older than 70 years of age indicated mean values of 1:8.5 and 1:13.1 with no sex-specific differences. These results are interpreted as pointing to a regressive activity of the pineal with advancing age (Meier and Gusek 1985). Entirely contradictory reports suggest significant pineal activity in old age. Tapp and Huxley (1972) found the pineal gland in the 75–90 years age-group to be 76–82% populated with pinealocytes without significant variation in the nuclear size. Studies on the pineal enzyme content also indicated lack of significant degeneration in old age (Wurtman et al. 1984).

The hypotensive effect of melatonin in humans in essential hypertension has been suggested (Birau 1981). The weight and volume of autopsied pineals in aging hypertensive patients were significantly greater than those of nonhypertensive patients. Hasegawa et al. (1987) examined aging human pineal weight and volume in 168 autopsy cases involving hypertensive and normotensive patients and concluded that human pineals do not degenerate after involution.

The Pineal Gland and Blindness

No significant histological differences were noted by Tapp (1979) between pineal glands from blind and normally sighted humans. Blindness causes early puberty, an effect opposite to that if the pineal were hyperactive in blind girls. Lehrer (1981) suggests that in blind humans and rats the pineal gland may contribute to longevity.

The Pineal Gland and Pregnancy

Morphological and biochemical changes in the pineal during pregnancy in humans and other animals have been reviewed briefly by Lew (1987). In these studies, increased activity in cytoplasmic organelles and pinealocyte enzymes during gestation was reported.

The Pineal Gland and Jet Lag

Human subjects were treated with a daily dose of 5 mg of melatonin in gelatin lactose for 3 days before flying back to London (eight time zones east) from a 14-day stay in San Francisco. The same preparation was taken for 4 days after reaching London. On day 7, the subjects rated their jet lag. It was found to be significantly less severe compared with those who were given a placebo (Arendt et al. 1986).

Pineal Morphology in Patients With Mood Disorders

Morphological investigations of the human pineal gland in patients suffering from various mood disorders, such as depression, have not been reported. Numerous pathological reports on the pineal in patients suffering from various physical and emotional disorders have not resulted in determining structure-disorder relationships. With the advent of highly sensitive melatonin bioassays (Ralph and Lynch 1970) and their continual refinements, highly accurate measurements of melatonin levels in human body fluids have become available. The link between pineal function and psychiatric disorders suspected for a long time has been established recently without a doubt (Demisch et al. 1987; Trentini et al. 1987; Waldhauser et al. 1984a, 1984b). Advances in the knowledge of morphological correlates of mood disorders remain to be established.

FUNCTIONS ATTRIBUTED TO THE PINEAL GLAND

As far as we know, one of the main functions of the pineal gland is the synthesis and secretion of melatonin. However, extrapineal tissues such as the retina, peripheral nerves, the harderian gland in rodents, enterochromaffin cells, and human erythrocytes (Vollrath 1981) also synthesize or secrete melatonin. Melatonin is also synthesized by rabbit platelets (Launay et al. 1982) and the rat hypothalamus and in the gastrointestinal tract. Synthesis of melatonin by pinealocytes may correspond to localized serotonin-producing argentaffin cells (Ebadi 1984). The chemical similarity of the melatonin synthesized by each of the above tissues remains to be determined. Numerous other substances besides melatonin have been identified within the mammalian pineal gland (see partial listing in Table 1-3).

Various functions have been ascribed to the pineal gland (Table 1-4). Some of these functions are well supported by data, whereas others are nothing but conjectures, speculations, and hypotheses. No target organ for pineal secretory products has yet been discovered. The morphological complexities of the pineal gland, its inaccessibility for experimental manipulations in animals, and the inability to pinpoint the morphological correlates of pineal secretory processes and secretory products contribute to our limited knowledge at present.

Table 1-4. Selective and partial listing of functions and roles ascribed to vertebrate pineal organ

ANECDOTAL, HISTORICAL
  Seat of the soul[a]
  Sphincter regulating flow of
    thought
  Appendix of the brain
  Penis cerebri
  Third eye

ANATOMICAL, MORPHOLOGICAL
  Conarium
  Endocrine gland
  Deep and superficial pineal
    regions discharging different
    functions
  Presence of cortex and medulla
  Pinealocyte as
    Neuron
    Paraneuron
    Pinealocyte I and II
    Pinealocyte sensu stricto (of
      several types)
    Dark, light pinealocytes
    Photoreceptor

Types of innervation
  Pinealofugal
    Sympathetic
    Parasympathetic
    Commissural (peptidergic)
  Pinealopetal
    to habenular nuclei

BIOCHEMICAL
  Enzyme clock
  Regulating center for biogenic
    amines
  (also see Table 1-3)

CLINICAL
  Diseases involving changes in
    pineal
    Carcinomas
    Epilepsy
    Hypertension
    Leprosy
    Muscular dystrophy
    Neurologic disorders
    Paget's disease
    Pinealitis
    Psychiatric disorders
    Psychosis

Table 1-4. Selective and partial listing of functions and roles ascribed to vertebrate pineal organ (continued)

Sexual disorders
Sexual precocity
Sudden infant death syndrome (SIDS)
Syphilis
Thyroid diseases
Tuberculosis
Tuberous sclerosis
Tumors
Tumorigenesis control; oncostatic
Use of pineal extracts (e.g., Epiphysan, Epiglandol, Epiphysormone) in treating disorders:
  Endocrine
  Genital
  Hypersexual
  Muscle inflammatory
  Neurologic
  Psychiatric
  Psychosis
    Juvenile
    Manic
    Puerperal
    Schizophrenia
  Tetanic
  Veterinary

Multipotentiality of pineal stem cells giving rise to
  Pigmented epithelial cells
  Lens cells
  Skeletal muscle fibers

ENVIRONMENTAL
External factors influencing pineal function:
  Darkness
  Irradiation
  Light (photic stimuli)
  Magnetism
  Noise, vibration
  Nutrition
  Olfaction
  Stress
  Temperature
Smaller pineals correlated with nocturnality
Larger pineals correlated with diurnality, endothermic species, and those living at high altitudes
Measures rainfall
Measures photoperiodic length
Independent magnetic sensor

DEVELOPMENTAL
Develops from two to three separate lobes
Composed of two genetically different parts (glandular and neuronal)

FICTITIOUS
Pineal calcification leading to a defective sense of direction (see note to Table 1-3)
Volvolon inducing muscular activity during sleep (see note to Table 1-3)

Table 1-4.   Selective and partial listing of functions and roles
ascribed to vertebrate pineal organ (continued)

HORMONAL
  Indoleamine synthesis
  Melatonin synthesis (see note to
    Table 1-3)

IMMUNOLOGICAL
  Provides immunity against stress

PHARMACOLOGICAL
  Pineal β-noradrenoceptors
    regulate *N*-acetyltransferase
    activity (NAT)
  Responds to pharmacological
    manipulations
  Tranquilizing organ

PHYSIOLOGICAL
  Amine precursor uptake and
    decarboxylation (APUD) cell
  Biological clock
  Breeding synchronizer
  Center for neurovegetative
    regulation
  Circadian neuroendocrine
    transducer
  Circadian rhythm controller
  Changes skin pigmentation
  "Communicates" with
    hypothalamus

Darkness or blinding increases
  pineal secretory activity
Endocrine gland
Endocrine-endocrine transducer
Influences
  Gonad development
  Pancreas
  Parathyroid
  Pituitary
  Suprarenal
  Thymus
  Thyroid
  All other endocrine glands
Inhibitor of other organ
  functions
Intermediary between
  environment (photoperiod)
  and endocrine system
Neuroendocrine transducer
Neurosecretory
Ovulation controller
Photoreception
Pineal secretion discharged into
  cerebrospinal fluid
Regulator of regulators
Seasonal breeding synchronizer
Sleep inducer
Thermoregulator

Note. This listing has been compiled from published sources. Citations
have been purposely avoided.
[a]René Descartes (1596–1650) or Cartesius is cited as the author of this
statement. However, according to Descartes, there is some organ in the
body in which the soul exerts its function more than in any other organ.
Such an organ was pineal as considered by Descartes (Kappers 1981).

REFERENCES

Abd-El-Basset EM, Kalnins VI, Subrahmanyan L, et al: 48-Kilodalton intermediate filament-associated protein in astrocytes. J Neurosci Res 19:1–13, 1988

Aguayo LG, Weight FF: Characterization of membrane currents in dissociated adult rat pineal cells. J Physiol (Lond) 405:397–419, 1988

Amendola BE, McClatchey K, Amendola MA: Pineal region tumors: analysis of treatment results. Int J Radiat Oncol Biol Phys 10:991–997, 1984

Arendt J, Aldhous M, Marks V: Alleviation of jet lag by melatonin: preliminary results of controlled double blind trial. Br Med J 292:1170, 1986

Bartsch C, Bartsch H: The biochemical events in the pineal gland during development (abstract), in International Workshop on Pineal Gland During Development (From Foetus to Adult). Neuroendocrinology Letters 7:152, 1985

Basinka J, Sastry PS, Stancer HC: Lipid composition of human, bovine and sheep pineal glands. J Neurochem 16:707–714, 1969

Bayliss CR, Bishop NL, Fowler RC: Pineal gland calcification and defective sense of direction. Br Med J 291:1758–1759, 1985 (see note to Table 1-3)

Bhatnagar KP: Ultrastructure of the pineal body of the common vampire bat, *Desmodus rotundus*. Am J Anat 181:163–178, 1988

Bhatnagar KP, Chang N, Merrell E: Ultrastructure of the pineal organ of the Indian mouse-tailed bat, *Rhinopoma microphyllum*. Myotis 23–24:45–49, 1985–1986

Bhatnagar KP, Frahm HD, Stephan H: The pineal organ of bats: a comparative morphological and volumetric investigation. J Anat 147:143–161, 1986

Bhatnagar KP, Frahm HD, Stephan H: The megachiropteran pineal organ: a comparative morphological and volumetric investigation with special emphasis on the remarkably large pineal of *Dobsonia praedatrix*. J Anat (in press)

Bignami A, Dahl D, Rueger DC: Glial fibrillary acidic (GFA) proteins in normal neural cells and in pathologic conditions. Advances in Cellular Neurobiology 1:285–310, 1980

Birau N: Melatonin in human serum: progress in screening investigation and clinic, in Melatonin—Current Status and Perspectives. Edited by Birau N, Schloot W. Oxford, Pergamon, 1981

Borit A, Schmidek HH: Pineal tumors and their treatment, in The Pineal Gland. Edited by Reiter RJ. New York, Raven, 1984

Bruckner R, Vorkapic P, Pendl G, et al: Pineal extirpation eliminates serum melatonin in patients with pineal tumors. J Neural Transm [Suppl] 21:495, 1986

Cardinali DP, Ritta MN: The role of prostaglandins in neuroendocrine junctions: studies in the pineal gland and the hypothalamus. Neuroendocrinology 36:152–160, 1983

Cardinali DP, Ritta MN, Vacas MI, et al: Molecular aspects of neuroendocrine integrative processes in the pineal gland, in The Pineal Gland and Its Endocrine Role. Edited by Axelrod J, Fraschini F, Velo GP. New York, Plenum, 1982

Chang N, Bhatnagar KP, Tseng MT, et al: Ultrastructure of the pineal gland of the tropical bat, *Rousettus leschenaulti*. Acta Anat (Basel) 128:194–203, 1987

Clarke JC: Computed tomography of pineal region ependymoma. Br J Radiol 61:953–955, 1988

Cohen M, Lippman M, Chabner B: Role of pineal gland in aetiology and treatment of breast cancer. Lancet 2:814–816, 1978

Collin JP, Oksche A: Structural and functional relationships in the nonmammalian pineal gland, in The Pineal Gland, Vol 1, Anatomy and Biochemistry. Edited by Reiter RJ. Boca Raton, FL, CRC Press, 1981

Commentz JC, Stahnke N, Stegner H, et al: Effects of cranial irradiation on pineal function in children with acute lymphatic leukemia (abstract), in International Workshop on Pineal Gland During Development (From Foetus to Adult). Neuroendocrinology Letters 7:145, 1985

Czarnocki J, Sastry PS, Stancer HC: The lipids in human pineal gland, in Biochemical Factors Concerned in the Functional Activity of the Nervous System. Edited by Richter D. London, Pergamon, 1969

Demisch L, Demisch K, Nickelsen T: Decrease of nocturnal melatonin in the plasmas of healthy adults following administration of dexamethasone, in Fundamentals and Clinics in Pineal Research. Edited by Trentini GP, De Gaetani C, Pévet P. New York, Raven, 1987

Diehl BJM: Occurrence and regional distribution of calcareous concretions in the rat pineal gland. Cell Tissue Res 195:359–366, 1978

Ebadi M: Regulation of the synthesis of melatonin and its significance to neuroendocrinology, in The Pineal Gland. Edited by Reiter RJ. New York, Raven, 1984, pp 1–37

Edmunds LN: Cellular and Molecular Bases of Biological Clocks: Models and Mechanisms for Circadian Timekeeping. Heidelberg, Springer, 1988

Eng LF, DeArmond SJ: Immunocytochemical studies of astrocytes in normal development and disease. Advances in Cellular Neurobiology 3:145–171, 1982

Futrell NN, Osborn AG, Cheson BD: Pineal region tumors: computed tomographic-pathologic spectrum. AJNR 2:415–420, 1981

Ganti SR, Hilal SK, Stein BM, et al: CT of pineal region tumors. AJNR 7:97–104, 1986

Gauquelin G, Geelen G, Allevard-Burguburn AM, et al: Presence of neurophysins I and II in the human pineal gland: comparison with the content of neurohypophyseal hormones. Peptides 3:805–809, 1982

Gudernatsch F: Miscellaneous organs, in Morris' Human Anatomy, 11th Edition. Edited by Schaeffer JP. New York, Blackiston, 1953

Gupta D: The pineal gland during development (abstract), in International Workshop on Pineal Gland During Development (From Foetus to Adult). Neuroendocrinology Letters 7:133, 1985

Hasegawa A, Ohtsubo K, Mori W: Pineal gland in old age: quantitative and qualitative morphological study of 168 human autopsy cases. Brain Res 409:343–349, 1987

Helmke K, Winkler P: Die Häufigkeit von Pinealisverkalkungen in den ersten 18 Lebensjahren. Fortschr Geb Rontgenstr Nuklearmed Erganzungsband 144:221–226, 1986

Hoffman HJ: Transcallosal approach to pineal tumors and the Hospital for Sick Children series of pineal region tumors, in Diagnosis and Treatment of Pineal Region Tumors. Edited by Neuwelt EA. Baltimore, MD, Williams & Wilkins, 1984

Hülsemann M: Vergleichende histologische Untersuchungen über das Vorkommen von Gliafasern in der Epiphysis cerebri von Säugetieren. Acta Anat (Basel) 66:249–278, 1967

Hülsemann M: Development of the innervation in the human pineal organ: light and electron microscopic investigations. Zeitschrift für Zellforschung und Mikroskopische Anatomie 115:396–415, 1971

Ichimura T, Arikuni T, Hashimoto PH: Fine-structural study of the pineal body of the monkey (*Macaca fuscata*) with special reference to synaptic formations. Cell Tissue Res 244:569–576, 1986

Iversen OH: Volvolon: a recently discovered peptide hormone from the pineal body. Can Med Assoc J 126:787–790, 1982 (see note to Table 1-3)

Kappers JA: A survey of advances in pineal research, in The Pineal Gland, Vol 1, Anatomy and Biochemistry. Edited by Reiter RJ. Boca Raton, FL, CRC Press, 1981

Karasek M: Functional ultrastructure of the mammalian pinealocyte, in Advances in Pineal Research, Vol 2. Edited by Reiter RJ, Fraschini F. London, Libbey, 1987

Kenny GCT, Scheelings FT: Observations of the pineal region of non-eutherian mammals. Cell Tissue Res 198:309–324, 1979

Kilgore DP, Strother CM, Starshak RJ, et al: Pineal germinoma: MR imaging. Radiology 158:435–438, 1986

King TS, Dougherty WJ: Effect of denervation on "synaptic" ribbon populations in the rat pineal gland. J Neurocytol 11:19–28, 1982

Kitay JI, Altschule MD: The Pineal Gland: A Review of the Physiologic Literature. Cambridge, MA, Harvard University Press, 1954

Korf HW, Oksche A, Ekström P, et al: Pinealocyte projections into the mammalian brain revealed with S-antigen antiserum. Science 231:735–737, 1986

Krstić R: Pineal calcification: its mechanism and significance. J Neural Transm [Suppl] 21:415–432, 1986

Landolt R, Hess HH: Regional distribution of some chemical structural components of the human nervous system, II: cerebrosides, proteolipid proteins and residue proteins. J Neurochem 13:1453–1459, 1966

Landolt R, Hess HH, Thalheimer C: Regional distribution of some chemical structural components of the human nervous system, I: DNA, RNA and ganglioside sialic acid. J Neurochem 13:1441–1452, 1966

Launay JM, Lemaitre BJ, Husson HP, et al: Melatonin synthesis by rabbit platelets. Life Sci 31:1487–1494, 1982

Legait H, Legait E: Contribution á l'étude de la glande pinéale humaine: étude faite á l'aide de 747 glandes. Bull Assoc Anat (Nancy) 61:107–121, 1977

Legait H, Bauchot R, Stephan H, et al: Etude des corrélations liant le volume de l'épiphyse aux poids somatique et encéphalique chez les rongeurs, les insectivores, les chiroptéres, les prosimiens et les simiens. Mammalia 40:327–337, 1976a

Legait H, Bauchot R, Contet-Audonneau JL: Etude des corrélations liant les volumes des lobes hypophysaires et de l'épiphyse au poids somatique et au poids encéphalique chez les chiroptéres. Bull Assoc Anat (Nancy) 60:175–188, 1976b

Lehrer S: Blindness increases life span of male rats: pineal effect on longevity. J Chronic Dis 34:427–429, 1981

Lehrer S, Levine E, Bloomner WD: Abnormally diminished sense of smell in women with oestrogen receptor positive breast cancer. Lancet 2:333, 1985

Lew GM: Morphological and biochemical changes in the pineal gland in pregnancy: minireview. Life Sci 41:2589–2596, 1987

Meier D, Gusek W: The pinealocytes' nucleocytoplasmic ratios of men of middle and advanced age (abstract), in International Workshop on Pineal Gland During Development (From Foetus to Adult). Neuroendocrinology Letters 7:137, 1985

Michotte Y, Lowenthal A, Knaepen L, et al: A morphological and chemical study of calcification of the pineal gland. Neurology 215:209–219, 1977

Miles A, Tidmarsch SF, Philbrick D, et al: Diagnostic potential of melatonin analysis in pineal tumors. N Engl J Med 313:329–330, 1985

Min KW, Seo IS, Song J: Postnatal evolution of the human pineal gland. Lab Invest 57:724–728, 1987

Møller M: The ultrastructure of the human fetal pineal gland, I: cell types and blood vessels. Cell Tissue Res 152:13–30, 1974

Møller M: The ultrastructure of the human fetal pineal gland, II: innervation and cell junctions. Cell Tissue Res 169:7–21, 1976

Møller M: Presence of a pineal nerve (nervus pinealis) in the human fetus: a light and electron microscopical study of the innervation of the pineal gland. Brain Res 154:1–12, 1978

O'Rahilly R: The development of the epiphysis cerebri and the subcommissural complex in staged human embryos (abstract). Anat Rec 160:488–489, 1968

Page TL: Transplantation of the cockroach circadian pacemaker. Science 216:73–75, 1982

Papasozomenos SCh: Glial fibrillary acidic (GFA) protein-containing cells in the human pineal gland. J Neuropathol Exp Neurol 42:391–408, 1983

Papasozomenos SCh: Pineal astrocytes, in Development, Morphology and Regional Specialization of Astrocytes, Vol 1. Edited by Fedoroff S, Vernadakis A. New York, Academic, 1986

Quay WB: Striated muscle in the mammalian pineal organ. Anat Rec 133:57–64, 1959

Quay WB: Histological structure and cytology of the pineal organ in birds and mammals, in Structure and Function of the Epiphysis Cerebri (Progress in Brain Research, Vol 10). Edited by Kappers JA, Schadé JP. Amsterdam, Elsevier, 1965

Quay WB: General biochemistry of the pineal gland of mammals, in The Pineal Gland, Vol 1, Anatomy and Biochemistry. Edited by Reiter RJ. Boca Raton, FL, CRC Press, 1981

Ralph CL: Pineal bodies and thermoregulation, in The Pineal Gland. Edited by Reiter RJ. New York, Raven, 1984

Ralph CL, Lynch HJ: A quantitative melatonin bioassay. Gen Comp Endocrinol 15:334–338, 1970

Reiter RJ (ed): The Pineal Gland. New York, Raven, 1984

Sack RL, Lewy AJ, Erb DL, et al: Human melatonin production decreases with age. J Pineal Res 3:379–388, 1986

Scharrer E: Photo-neuro-endocrine systems: general concepts. Ann N Y Acad Sci 117:13–22, 1964

Sparks DL, Hunsaker JC III: The pineal gland in sudden infant death syndrome: preliminary observations. J Pineal Res 5:111–118, 1988

Takahashi JS, Menaker M: Multiple redundant circadian oscillators within the isolated avian pineal gland. J Comp Physiol [A] 154:435–440, 1984

Tapp E: The histology and pathology of the human pineal gland, in The Pineal Gland of Vertebrates Including Man (Progress in Brain Research, Vol 52). Edited by Kappers JA, Pévet P. Amsterdam, Elsevier, 1979

Tapp E: The histological appearances of the pineal gland from puberty to old age, in The Pineal Gland During Development: From Fetus to Adult. Edited by Gupta D, Reiter RJ. London, Croom Helm, 1986, pp 89–99

Tapp E, Huxley M: The histological appearance of the human pineal gland from puberty to old age. Journal of Pathology and Bacteriology 108:137–144, 1972

Taylor CM, McLaughlin B, Weiss JB: Bovine and human pineal glands contain substantial quantities of endothelial cell stimulating angiogenic factor. J Neural Transm 71:79–84, 1988

Trentini GP, De Gaetani CF, Pierini G, et al: Some aspects of human pineal pathology, in Advances in Pineal Research. Edited by Reiter RJ, Karasek M. London, Libbey, 1986

Trentini GP, De Gaetani C, Pévet P (eds): Fundamentals and Clinics in Pineal Research. New York, Raven, 1987

Vollrath L: Comparative morphology of the vertebrate pineal complex, in The Pineal Gland of Vertebrates Including Man (Progress in Brain Research, Vol 52). Edited by Kappers JA, Pévet P. Amsterdam, Elsevier, 1979

Vollrath L: The Pineal Organ, in Handbuch der mikroskopischen Anatomie des Menschen, Vol VI/7. Edited by Oksche A, Vollrath L. Berlin, Springer, 1981

Vollrath L: Functional anatomy of the human pineal gland, in The Pineal Gland. Edited by Reiter RJ. New York, Raven, 1984

Von Eyl O, Gusek W: Zur Frage von Altersveränderungen der Zirbelddrüse beim Menschen. Verh Dtsch Ges Pathol 59:400–404, 1975

Vorkapic P, Pendl G: Microsurgery of pineal region lesions in children. Neuropediatrics 18:222–226, 1987

Waldhauser F, Gisinger B: The pineal gland and its development in human puberty, in The Pineal Gland During Development: From Fetus to Adult. Edited by Gupta D, Reiter RJ. London, Croom Helm, 1986, pp 134–143

Waldhauser F, Weissenbacher G, Zeitlhuber U, et al: Fall in nocturnal serum melatonin levels during prepuberty and pubescence. Lancet 1:362–365, 1984a

Waldhauser F, Lynch HJ, Wurtman RJ: Melatonin in human body fluids: clinical significance, in The Pineal Gland. Edited by Reiter RJ. New York, Raven, 1984b

Waldhauser F, Steger H, Vorkapic P: Melatonin secretion in man and the influence of exogenous melatonin on some physiological and behavioural variables, in Advances in Pineal Research, Vol 2. Edited by Reiter RJ, Fraschini F. London, Libbey, 1987

Walls EW: The blood vascular and lymphatic systems, in Cunningham's Text Book of Anatomy, 10th Edition. Edited by Romanes GJ. London, Oxford, 1964

Wartenberg H: The mammalian pineal organ: electron microscopic studies on the fine structure of pinealocytes, glial cells and on the perivascular compartment. Zeitschrift für Zellforschung and Mikroskopische Anatomie 86:78–97, 1968

Wetterberg L: Melatonin in psychiatric conditions, in Melatonin—Current Status and Perspectives. Edited by Birau N, Schloot W. New York, Pergamon, 1981

Wiechman AF, Bok D, Horwitz J: Localization of hydroxyindole-O-methyltransferase in the mammalian pineal gland and retina. Invest Ophthalmol Vis Sci 26:253–265, 1985

Wurtman RJ, Axelrod J, Kelly DE: The Pineal. New York, Academic, 1968

Wurtman RJ, Axelrod J, Barchas JD: Age and enzyme activity in the human pineal. Endocrinology 24:299–301, 1984

Zimmerman RA, Bilaniuk LT: Age-related incidence of pineal calcification detected by computed tomography. Radiology 142:659–661, 1982

Chapter 2

Pineal Rhythmicity: Neural, Behavioral, and Endocrine Consequences

Russel J. Reiter, Ph.D.

Chapter 2

Pineal Rhythmicity: Neural, Behavioral, and Endocrine Consequences

Perhaps more effectively than any other group of clinicians, psychiatrists have incorporated basic information about the function of the pineal gland into the clinical setting. Information accumulated to date clearly implicates the pineal gland and its chief hormonal constituent, melatonin, in a variety of psychiatric disorders. Much of this information will be reviewed in subsequent chapters. The purpose of this chapter is to summarize the rhythmic nature of pineal functions in mammals, including humans, and briefly describe how this information may have an impact on affective and related behaviors. The pineal gland of all mammals exhibits obvious circadian rhythms that may influence behavior during any 24-hour period. Additionally, seasonal rhythms in mood tentatively have been linked to circannual fluctuations in pineal physiology.

RHYTHMS IN NERVE ENDINGS WITHIN THE PINEAL GLAND

The sympathetic innervation of the mammalian pineal gland is absolutely essential for the rhythmic function of this organ. Postganglionic sympathetic fibers whose cell bodies are located in the superior cervical ganglia innervate the pineal and terminate in the vicinity of pinealocytes, the endocrine units of the gland. The superior cervical ganglia receive information about the photoperiodic environment by way of a complex pathway that involves ganglion cells of the retinas, neurons in the suprachiasmatic nucleus (SCN) of the anterobasal hypothalamus, and intermediolateral cell column neurons in the upper thoracic cord; these latter cells provide the preganglionic sympathetic connections to the superior cervical ganglia. Besides the

Work by R.J.R. was supported by grants from NSF and NIH.

obviously important peripheral sympathetic innervation to the pineal, the gland also receives centripetal fibers, directly via its stalk, from the central nervous system (Korf and Møller 1984); the functional impact of these fibers, if any, on the biosynthetic and/or secretory activity of the pineal gland remains unknown (see Figure 2-1).

The chief, but perhaps not the only, neurotransmitter released from the postganglionic sympathetic fibers onto the pinealocytes is norepinephrine (NE) (Zatz 1981). The discharge of NE from these fibers is initiated by action potentials that are generated by electrical activity originating in the SCN. In general, during the daily dark period, the SCN, due to its presumed intrinsic electrical activity, induces the release of NE from the sympathetic fibers in the pineal gland. During the day, light acting on the retinas suppresses the activity of the SCN and thereby diminishes the discharge of NE from

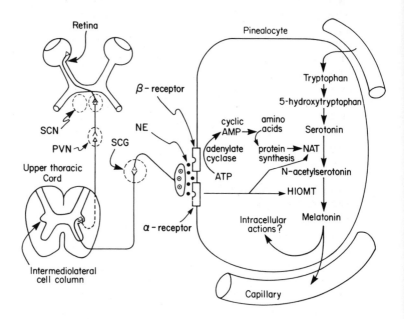

Figure 2-1. Neural connections between eyes and pineal gland as demonstrated in various mammals and synthesis of melatonin within pineal gland. HIOMT, hydroxyindole-O-methyltransferase; NAT, N-acetyltransferase; NE, norepinephrine; PVN, paraventricular nucleus; SCG, superior cervical ganglia; SCN, suprachiasmatic nucleii.

postganglionic fibers in the pineal gland. Thus, in general, the pineal gland is normally activated during darkness, and its activity is suppressed during the day. Clearly, the circadian rhythms in the pineal gland are governed by the 24-hour cycle of light and darkness and the associated alteration in the number of action potentials arriving in the pineal gland via its sympathetic innervation.

The actual measurements of the 24-hour variations in the NE content of the nerve endings in the pineal gland reveal that in some species, e.g., the rat, a circadian rhythm exists, with highest levels of the catecholamine being present during the night when the gland is most active (Wurtman and Axelrod 1974). In contrast, in neither the Syrian hamster or the cotton rat (*Sigmodon hispidus*) does the pineal content of NE over a 24-hour period change. However, metabolic studies of catecholamine production clearly indicate that, in all mammalian species examined, NE production in pineal nerve endings increases during the night. The index used as a basis for this judgment is the activity of the enzyme tyrosine hydroxylase (TH), the rate-limiting enzyme in catecholamine production. TH converts tyrosine to dopa in sympathetic nerve endings; dopa is then decarboxylated by the enzyme dopa decarboxylase. When the activity of this latter enzyme is pharmacologically inhibited, dopa accumulates in proportion to TH activity. In the case of the mammalian pineal gland, studies indicate that catecholamine production (including NE) is significantly greater at night than during the day (Craft et al. 1984). Thus, the production of the neurotransmitter that promotes the biosynthetic activity within the pinealocytes is greater at night than during the day.

The nocturnal increase in the electrical activity of the pineal postganglionic sympathetic nerves not only induces the increased production of the neurotransmitter NE but also initiates its release into the postsynaptic cleft. Other neurotransmitters or neuromodulators may also be present in the same vesicular compartment in the nerve endings and thereby may be released concomitantly with NE; possible substances that fall into this category include serotonin and neuropeptide Y, among others.

RHYTHMS WITHIN THE PINEALOCYTE

As at other sites, released NE in the pineal gland is subjected to various fates. Thus, it can be taken up by the neurons from which it was released, diffuse away from the site of its release, be metabolized locally, or bind to receptors on the pinealocyte membrane. This latter activity is of obvious interest to pinealogists, because the nocturnal activity of the pinealocyte unequivocally depends on NE discharged from the sympathetic nerve endings.

Membrane Adrenergic Receptors

NE acts on both β- and α-adrenergic receptors, and both have been localized in the pinealocyte membrane. In the case of melatonin production within the pineal gland, however, the action of NE primarily depends on its interaction with β-adrenergic receptors (Klein 1985; Morgan et al. 1988; Zatz 1981). Hence, the administration of propranolol, a β-receptor antagonist, essentially totally blocks the nocturnal increase in pineal melatonin production in animals, as well as the nighttime rise in circulating melatonin in humans. Antagonists that interfere with α-adrenergic receptors have only a minor influence on the ability of the pineal gland to produce melatonin at night.

Pharmacologically, melatonin production can be induced in the pineal gland of many species by the administration of the endogenous neurotransmitter NE or by injecting the specific β-receptor agonist isoproterenol. The efficacy of NE in such experiments is greatly enhanced if the neurotransmitter is given in conjunction with a reuptake blocker, e.g., imipramine. Because of an active reuptake system by the postganglionic sympathetic fibers that innervate the pineal gland, the pinealocytes may be protected from circulating (either exogenously administered or endogenously produced, such as during stress) catecholamines. This problem is circumvented when isoproterenol is used, because it is not taken up by sympathetic nerve endings.

The responsiveness of the pinealocytes to NE or isoproterenol varies greatly among species. In the rat and Djungarian hamster, β-receptor agonists are capable of promoting pineal melatonin production either during the day or at night, i.e., throughout the 24-hour period (Steinlechner et al. 1985; Vaughan et al. 1986). However, in the Syrian hamster, β-adrenergic receptor agonists are effective as melatonin-stimulating agents only for a brief interval late in the dark phase of the light-dark cycle. Thus, there is a striking circadian variation in the sensitivity of the Syrian hamster pineal gland (in terms of melatonin production) to NE or isoproterenol. Such a circadian rhythm of sensitivity may also be operative in humans because the infusion of isoproterenol to humans during the day does not, as in Syrian hamsters, promote high circulating melatonin titers. Similar studies on humans have not been conducted at night, when the Syrian hamster pineal gland is known to exhibit a marked rise in melatonin production in response to β-adrenergically active substances.

Numerous β-adrenergic receptor ligands have been used to determine the 24-hour rhythms of these receptors on pinealocyte membranes. In those species in which thorough studies have been conducted, obvious 24-hour rhythms in the number of pinealocyte β-receptors have been uncovered. However, the rhythms exhibited vary among species and the number of receptors on the pinealocyte membrane do not parallel the sensitivity of the pinealocytes (in terms of melatonin synthesis) to the β-receptor agonists.

Whereas several reports showed 24-hour variations in the number of β-receptors on rat pinealocytes, the phasing of the rhythms varies; recent studies have yielded more consistent data that have also been found to have a physiological basis. With use of radioactive iodocyanopindolol (ICYP), a nighttime increase in the number of β-adrenergic receptors on rat pinealocyte membranes was observed in sexually immature and mature rats, with the rise in the number of receptors occurring near the time of the endogenous melatonin peak (Reiter et al. 1985). This and other reports also show that β-receptors are available on the rat pinealocyte during the day, presumably accounting for the daytime and nighttime sensitivity of the rat pineal gland to β-adrenergic stimulation (Zatz et al. 1976).

With an even more specific ligand, i.e., iodopindolol, the nighttime rise in the number of β-receptors on the rat pinealocyte membrane was confirmed by Gonzalez-Brito et al. (1988a). Furthermore, this group found that the rhythm in the receptors could be modified either by changing the release of NE from the sympathetic nerve endings within the pineal gland by light exposure or by blocking the binding of NE to the pinealocyte receptor by propranolol administration (Gonzalez-Brito et al. 1988b). From their physiological studies, it is apparent that the release of NE from pineal sympathetic neurons at night eventually desensitizes (downregulates?) the receptors on the pinealocyte membrane (Gonzalez-Brito et al. 1988b). During the day, when NE release is low, and during the early dark period, the receptors are again upregulated so that when endogenous NE is released, maximum melatonin production occurs. Recall, however, that in the rat pineal, melatonin production is responsive to β-receptor agonists even during the light phase of the light-dark cycle.

β-Receptors on the Syrian hamster pinealocyte membrane also exhibit a 24-hour variation (Pangerl et al. 1989). In this species, unlike in the rat, pineal gland melatonin production can be induced by β-receptor agonists for a short interval during the daily dark period (Reiter et al. 1987b). One potential explanation for the lack of responsiveness of the hamster and human pineal gland to drugs such as isoproterenol during the day would be the lack of β-adrenergic receptors on the pinealocyte membrane. When measured over a 24-hour period with iodopindolol as the receptor ligand, it was in fact found that during the light phase of the light-dark cycle, ligand binding was very robust, proving the availability of numerous β-adrenergic receptors on the hamster pinealocyte membrane (Pangerl et al. 1989). During the night, when NE is released from the sympathetic neurons innervating the pineal gland, melatonin production is stimulated and the receptors are subsequently downregulated. Shortly after reaching their nadir, the receptors are rapidly upregulated and, therefore, already abundantly available during the early morning hours and, in fact, throughout the day. Hence, the lack of β-receptors is not an explanation for the inability of the Syrian hamster pineal gland to form melatonin during the day. Subsequent studies have shown that the concentration of cyclic AMP (cAMP), the second messenger in the stimulation of melatonin production, is increased after β-receptor agonist administration during both the day and the night (C. Santana, J.M. Guerrero, R.J.R., unpublished observations). This implies that a post-cAMP mechanism limits melatonin production in the pineal gland in this species to a very brief period late in the dark phase.

The information that has accumulated on the control of melatonin production in the Syrian hamster pineal gland may be applicable to humans. In the human, as in the Syrian hamster, isoproterenol infusion during the day was not found to be associated with a rise in circulating melatonin (Vaughan et al. 1976). Yet, the endogenous rise in blood melatonin titers is blocked by propranolol. Perhaps in the human pineal as well, daytime melatonin production and release are limited by a post-cAMP mechanism.

To date, there are no studies on β-adrenergic receptors in the human pineal gland. Presumably, they would exhibit a circadian rhythm that would be linked to endogenously released NE from the intrapineal sympathetic nerve endings as has been found in other mammals. Besides NE release from the nerve endings that terminate in the pineal gland, circulating catecholamines from the adrenal medulla and other nerve terminals could influence the number of pineal β-receptors, as well as the activity of the pineal gland. Studies of this type have been common in nonhuman mammals, but are rare in humans (Reiter 1988).

α-Adrenergic receptors have also been identified from membranes recovered from rat (Vacas et al. 1980) and Syrian hamster (A. Pangerl, B. Pangerl, R.J.R., unpublished observations) pineal glands. At least in the rat, the α-receptors do not exhibit a 24-hour rhythm. As noted above, these receptors are also acted on by NE and serve to augment the melatonin response to β-adrenergic receptor stimulation. Whether α-adrenergic receptors exist in human pineal tissue has not been satisfactorily determined.

cAMP Concentrations

β-Adrenergic receptors are linked to the enzyme adenylate cyclase by guanosine-binding protein (G protein). The interaction of NE with the β-receptor thus results in a stimulation of adenylate cyclase with the resultant conversion of ATP to the intracellular messenger, adenosine $3'$-,$5'$-monophosphate, or cAMP (Strada et al. 1972). Because NE is normally released from the pineal nerve endings at night, it is expected that the cAMP concentrations would likewise be highest at this time. Although α-adrenergic stimulation of the rat pinealocyte may further promote cAMP levels induced by β_1-adrenergic receptor stimulation, the stimulation of the a_1-receptors alone does not promote cAMP accumulation in cultured glands (Vanecek et al. 1985). Whether there are actually 24-hour rhythms of cAMP concentrations in the pineal gland of the rat remains unknown, although the response of this constituent to exogenously administered isoproterenol does vary with time of day.

Phosphodiesterase normally metabolizes cAMP; a change in the activity of this enzyme over a 24-hour period could generate a circadian rhythm in the concentration of the cyclic nucleotide. The 24-hour levels of pineal phosphodiesterase activity remain uninvestigated in experimental animals.

Serotonin Concentrations

Serotonin concentrations in the mammalian pineal gland are higher than in any other organ tested (Giarman and Day 1959). Pineal serotonin is acted on by numerous enzymes; thus, it may be oxidatively deaminated to 5-hydroxyindole acetaldehyde, N-acetylated to N-acetylserotonin, or O-methylated to 5-methoxytryptamine. Each of these conversions, in addition to its rate of synthesis, may well be instrumental in determining the pineal levels of serotonin over a 24-hour period. Usually, daytime concentrations of pineal serotonin are greater than those measured at night (rat, Quay 1963; Syrian hamster, Steinlechner et al. 1985; cotton rat, Matthews et al. 1982; Richardson's ground squirrel, Reiter et al. 1984). Because serotonin is actively N-acetylated in the pineal gland at night, as will be seen in a subsequent section, it is widely believed that this conversion primarily accounts for the nighttime reduction in serotonin levels. Despite the general acceptance of this conclusion, some data are incompatible with this simplified explanation of the pineal serotonin rhythm (King et al. 1984b).

Besides its differential metabolism throughout the light-dark cycle, the synthesis of pineal serotonin also exhibits a 24-hour rhythm. Here, again, there are species differences. In the rat, maximal pineal serotonin production occurs coincidentally with its maximum metabolism, i.e., at night. On the other hand, in the pineal gland of the Syrian hamster, serotonin is most abundantly produced during the daytime (King et al. 1984a; Steinlechner et al. 1983). In view of this, the generation of the serotonin rhythms may differ in the rat and Syrian hamster pineal gland. High quantities of serotonin are also found in the human pineal gland, but little is known as to what regulates the concentration of serotonin.

N-Acetyltransferase Activity

The conversion of serotonin, a major constituent of the pineal gland, to melatonin is a two-step process. Initially, serotonin is N-acetylated by the enzyme serotonin N-acetyltransferase (NAT) to produce N-acetylserotonin; this compound is subsequently O-methylated by the enzyme hydroxyindole-O-methyltransferase (HIOMT) with the subsequent production of N1-acetyl-5-methoxytryptamine, commonly known as melatonin (Ebadi 1984) (Figure 2-2). NAT activity correlates closely with melatonin production under many circumstances (Wilkinson et al. 1977), and, under most conditions, the N-acetylation of serotonin seems to be rate limiting in melatonin production (Ebadi 1984).

Typically, the increased NE stimulation of the pinealocyte during darkness is associated with a commensurate rise in NAT activity (Klein and Weller 1970). However, among mammals the magnitude of the nighttime increase in NAT activity varies widely (Rudeen et al. 1975). Of the animals investigated, the rat exhibits the greatest nocturnal rise (50–100 times minimal daytime levels) in the activity of the acetylating enzyme. In contrast, in the guinea pig pineal, NAT activity only doubles at night. There may be some species and/or some circumstances under which a pineal NAT rhythm is intermittently absent (Reiter et al. 1987a).

The control of the circadian rhythm in NAT activity and, thus, melatonin production has been widely investigated in the rat and the Syrian hamster pineal gland. The nocturnal rise in NAT activity is induced by cAMP-dependent protein kinase activity and requires the synthesis of new protein and nRNA (Guerrero et al. 1988; Weiss and Strada 1972). Whether the newly produced protein is actually the

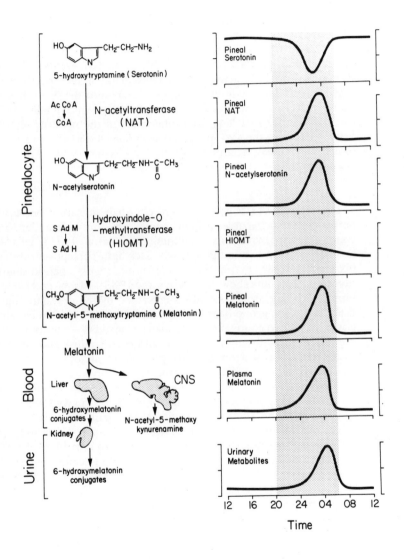

Figure 2-2. Rhythms in various pineal, blood, and urinary constituents as known to exist in mammals, including humans.

enzyme NAT or whether it is another molecule that then secondarily induces the enzyme remains undetermined.

Although in the rat and the Syrian hamster a nocturnal increase in NAT activity is observed, the pattern of the rise differs. In the rat, NAT activity typically increases gradually beginning with the onset of darkness and reaches a peak at roughly middarkness (Ebadi 1984). By comparison, NAT activity in the pineal gland of the Syrian hamster remains near daytime levels for several hours into the dark phase; it then rapidly rises to reach a short-term peak after which it falls quickly (Steinlechner et al. 1984). The differences in the patterns of NAT activity between the two species are also reflected in their nocturnal patterns of pineal melatonin production (Reiter 1986). The NAT rhythm in the human pineal gland is presumably similar to that in the rat, inasmuch as the human blood melatonin rhythm is reminiscent of that in the rat.

The pineal NAT rhythm is truly circadian in nature because it persists in rats incapable of light perception, although under these conditions the rhythm is free-running (Klein et al. 1971). This also holds for humans—blind people who lack light perception exhibit a plasma melatonin rhythm that is free-running with a period slightly exceeding 24 hours (Lewy and Newsome 1983). In rats, and likely in humans, the melatonin rhythm is entrained by the prevailing light-dark cycle. One group has proposed that the rat pineal NAT cycle is governed by two endogenous circadian pacemakers—one controlling the onset of nocturnal NAT activity and cued to dusk and a second linked to dawn that determines the drop in activity of the acetylating enzyme (Illnerová 1988). A contrasting theory assumes that one pacemaker governs both the onset and offset of the activity of the serotonin-acetylating enzyme in the pineal gland (Lewy 1985).

The nighttime rise in serotonin N-acetylation causes a pineal increase in the product of this conversion, i.e., N-acetylserotonin. The melatonin-forming enzyme, HIOMT, although initially reported to exhibit a 24-hour rhythm (Wurtman et al. 1963), seems not to when more sensitive methods are used for its measurement (Ebadi 1984). Because HIOMT activity is high in the pineal, by mass action N-acetylserotonin is converted to melatonin.

Melatonin Concentrations

A 24-hour fluctuation (high levels at night, low levels during the day) in pineal melatonin content is a characteristic of almost all mammals (Reiter 1987a). High nighttime pineal melatonin is found in both nocturnally active and diurnally active animals and in those species that exhibit a crepuscular pattern of locomotor activity, i.e., activity concentrated at the light-to-dark or dark-to-light transitions. At least one species, the domestic pig (*Sus scrofa*), may seasonally lack a circadian pineal melatonin rhythm (Reiter et al. 1987a). Certain inbred strains of mice reportedly lack the genetic machinery required for the expression of either NAT or HIOMT, and, therefore, they likewise are devoid of a 24-hour pineal melatonin cycle (Ebihara et al. 1986).

Whereas a nocturnal rise in pineal melatonin concentration is typical, the pattern and the duration of the night-associated elevated melatonin seems to vary among species. Thus, three patterns of nighttime melatonin have been provisionally described (Reiter 1987a), although the significance, if any, of a particular pattern remains unknown. It seems universally true, however, that if the ratio of light to darkness during a 24-hour period is changed to favor darkness, elevated pineal melatonin levels are prolonged. This is one means by which the pineal gland, via the secretion of melatonin, could signal the animal as to the approaching seasons. It is, of course, well known that many seasonal aspects of physiology, including reproduction, in animals under natural photoperiods are determined by the circannual fluctuations in day length, which, in turn, alter melatonin secretion and thereby endocrine physiology (Reiter 1980).

As noted above, if animals (Reiter et al. 1971) or humans (Lewy and Newsome 1983) are incapable of perceiving light by way of the eyes, the pineal melatonin rhythm persists but is free-running, and, as a consequence, it is not in synchrony with the prevailing light-dark environment. In surgically blinded rats, peak pineal melatonin concentrations occur coincidentally with the greatest locomotor activity of the animal (Reiter et al. 1971). In one blind human, the free-running period of the plasma melatonin cycle was calculated to be 24.7 hours (Lewy and Newsome 1983).

RHYTHMS OF MELATONIN IN BODY FLUIDS

Little is known concerning the secretion of melatonin from the pinealocyte. It is generally agreed that melatonin is not stored for any length of time within the pineal gland. Rather, once produced, it is presumed that it rapidly diffuses from the cell. Because of melatonin's high lipid solubility, the cell membrane of not only the pinealocyte but of other organs as well seems to provide little impediment to its passage. Although large quantities of melatonin seem not to be stored for any appreciable time in the pineal, its discharge from the cell can seemingly be experimentally hastened. Thus, short-duration forced swimming in experimental animals when pineal melatonin levels are high seems to cause a rapid depletion of pineal melatonin in spite of continued high synthesis of the indole, i.e., elevated NAT activity (Troiani et al. 1988).

There are several potential routes of secretion of melatonin. Although most investigators accept the discharge of melatonin into the blood vascular system (Rollag et al. 1978), its direct secretion into the cerebrospinal fluid (CSF) remains a possibility.

Blood

The rhythmic production of melatonin in the pineal gland is paralleled by similar changes in the concentration of this constituent in the blood (Wilkinson et al. 1977). Even though a number of other organs are known to produce melatonin (Pang and Allen 1986), surgical removal of the pineal gland eliminates the nighttime rise in circulating melatonin titers in experimental animals (Lewy et al. 1980; Vaughan and Reiter 1986) and in humans (Neuwelt and Lewy 1983).

Details regarding the cycles of melatonin in the blood are not as clear as they are for pineal concentrations of the constituent (Reiter 1986). It is apparent, however, that in all animals the blood melatonin rhythm is very stable, i.e., not easily perturbed. This is a state that would be expected of a rhythm that is an important time regulator to the organism, a function the melatonin signal may well provide (Armstrong et al. 1986). The stability of the melatonin rhythm has been noted in humans as well. Although rarely put into print, investigators in the area agree that measurement of the circadian blood melatonin rhythm in a subject at different times results in cycles that are virtually superimposable.

The human plasma melatonin cycle was first described in 1973 by Pelham and colleagues with a highly specific, but relatively insensitive, bioassay. The rhythm subsequently has been defined in greater detail with more sensitive techniques such as gas chromatography–mass spectrometry (Lewy et al. 1980) and radioimmunoassay (Arendt 1985; Vaughan 1984). In humans, as in experimental animals, drugs that interfere with the action of NE on β-adrenergic receptors also modify circulating melatonin levels, presumably because they decrease the pineal synthesis and/or release of melatonin (Vaughan et al. 1976; Wetterberg 1978). The human melatonin rhythm may change with the seasons (Arendt et al. 1979), with menstrual cyclicity (Hariharasubramanian et al. 1986), and certainly with age (Iguchi et al. 1982) (see Chapter 7). In the latter case, attenuation of the plasma melatonin cycle is seen. Additionally in humans, puberty may be associated with a substantial drop in nighttime melatonin titers, a change hypothesized to be permissive to normal pubertal development (Waldhauser and Steger 1986).

Cerebrospinal Fluid

Melatonin in the blood rapidly passes through the choroid plexus and into the CSF of animals and presumably humans. The possibility exists for a direct release of melatonin from the pineal into the CSF in those species in which a subcollosal, as opposed to a supracollosal, pineal gland exists. Although a direct discharge of melatonin into the CSF has been proposed, this concept is not generally widely accepted (Reiter 1987b).

The first complete study on CSF melatonin levels over a 24-hour light-dark regimen was carried out by Hedlund et al. (1977) in calves. They reported a very conspicuous variation, with highest melatonin levels being detected, as in the blood, during the dark phase of the light-dark environment. In this study, they compared plasma and CSF concentrations of melatonin and actually found higher titers in the ventricle, a difference that remains unexplained.

The only other species in which CSF melatonin levels have been thoroughly examined is the rhesus monkey (Reppert et al. 1980). As in the calf, a high-magnitude melatonin cycle with low values during the day is also apparent in this species. The CSF melatonin rhythm is obliterated by continual light exposure, but persists in continual darkness (Perlow et al. 1980). Finally, inverting the light-dark cycle also phase shifted the CSF melatonin rhythm in the monkey (Reppert et al. 1981). The findings are consistent with the CSF melatonin rhythm being endogenous and normally synchronized by the light-dark environment.

Although melatonin has been identified in the CSF of humans, little is known of its circadian rhythmicity (Vaughan 1984). On the other hand, considering what is known of CSF melatonin concentrations over a 24-hour period in other mammalian species, it seems likely that in humans a similar rhythm of ventricular fluid melatonin exists. Whether melatonin in the CSF is functionally more or less important than melatonin in the blood must await future experimentation.

Saliva

Wetterberg (1979) was the first to detect melatonin in human saliva, whereas its circadian fluctuation in this fluid was left to Miles et al. (1985) and Vakkuri (1985). A comparison of blood and salivary melatonin levels indicates that the values in saliva are about one-third those in the blood; however, the melatonin rhythms in the two fluids are very similar, suggesting that melatonin in the blood readily passes through the secretory cells of the salivary glands. If salivary melatonin levels are to be reliably monitored, there are certain restrictions in terms of what subjects can eat immediately before saliva collection. On the other hand, salivary melatonin levels represent a convenient, noninvasive means of monitoring pineal activity in humans and other large mammals. Other than for humans, there are no data on salivary melatonin concentrations.

Exposure of subjects to bright light at night when blood and salivary melatonin levels are high causes the expected and parallel drop in melatonin in both fluids (McIntyre et al. 1987). When patients are returned to darkness after 1 hour of light exposure, melatonin levels rise in a parallel fashion. These findings suggest the dependence of salivary concentrations of melatonin on the circulating titers of the constituent.

FACTORS THAT PERTURB MELATONIN RHYTHMICITY

The point has already been made that the melatonin cycle seems to be highly stable. For example, it is difficult to perturb the rhythm with endocrine manipulations or nutritional modifications. On the other hand, light (Reiter 1985) and, to a much lesser degree, stress (or exercise) (Reiter 1988) have a significant impact on circadian melatonin production.

Light Intensity

The imposition of light during the normal dark period when melatonin levels in the pineal gland and blood are elevated leads to a rapid decline in the concentrations of the indole. Particularly within the pineal gland, melatonin content drops precipitously after light exposure at night. For example, in the cotton rat, pineal melatonin values are reduced by 50% within 2 minutes after the onset of light at night (Thiele et al. 1983). In all species tested, the t½ (half-time) for light suppression of pineal melatonin content is less than 10 minutes (Brainard et al. 1982; Reiter et al. 1983; Rollag et al. 1980). The cessation of melatonin production most likely accounts for the drop in levels within the gland. With light onset, the electrical activity of the SCN is immediately inhibited; this reduces the release of NE from the sympathetic nerve endings in the pineal gland, and, as a consequence, the intrapinealocyte machinery governing melatonin synthesis is shut off, leading to the reduction in the quantity of the indole in the cells. Even when the light exposure is very brief (e.g., 1 second) at night, pineal melatonin levels are depressed to basal daytime values 30 minutes later (Reiter et al. 1986).

Whereas light readily suppressed pineal melatonin production in those mammalian species in which it has been examined, the light intensity (irradiance) required to interrupt melatonin synthesis varies greatly among species. Thus, the effect intensities of light vary from $0.0005 \ \mu W/cm^2$ for the albino rat (Webb et al. 1985) to roughly $1850 \ \mu W/cm^2$ for the Richardson's ground squirrel (Reiter et al. 1983). The human pineal gland responds to light at an intensity intermediate between these two values. In general, the pineal gland of diurnally active species seems somewhat less sensitive to light inhibition than does the pineal of nocturnally active rodents (Reiter 1985). Preliminary studies suggest that, at least in the Djungarian hamster, the ability of acute light exposure at night to suppress pineal melatonin production may relate to the ambient temperature to which the animals are exposed; thus, reducing the temperature seems to decrease the responsiveness of the pineal gland to light exposure (Steinlechner et al. 1988).

Light suppression of pineal melatonin production in mammals seems to be an all-or-nothing response (Reiter 1985), although in humans it may be a graded reduction with increasing light intensity, judging from the changes in plasma melatonin levels (McIntyre et al. 1987).

Light Wavelength

Besides the brightness of light, the wavelength (color) of light to which animals or humans are exposed may be instrumental in determining the ability of the pineal gland to convert serotonin to melatonin (Reiter 1985). In Syrian hamsters (Brainard et al. 1984) and humans (Brainard et al. 1985), blue light wavelengths (approximately 500–520 mm) seem to be most suppressive to melatonin. This suggests, but certainly does not prove, that rhodopsin may be the photopigment that mediates the inhibitory effect of light on pineal melatonin synthesis. The findings have clear implications for phototherapy in humans.

PHYSIOLOGICAL CONSEQUENCES OF MELATONIN

Behavioral and Neural Effects

Melatonin administration to experimental animals has a variety of neurochemical effects, although many of these have not been definitively characterized. The administration of this indole to rats reportedly increases brain stem serotonin levels (Anton-Tay et al. 1968). This neurotransmitter has been implicated in sleep mechanisms;

another of melatonin's actions is that of inducing sleepiness in humans (Anton-Tay et al. 1971; Cramer et al. 1974; Vollrath et al. 1975). Perhaps the great attenuation of the melatonin rhythm in humans with advanced age may be in part responsible for the general deterioration in sleep efficiency in older individuals. If this is proven to be true, melatonin may have utility in the improvement of sleep quality for these individuals. Melatonin also prolongs the intervals required for experimental animals to recover from barbital-induced anesthesia. These and other neural effects of melatonin have been summarized elsewhere (Reiter 1977; Wurtman and Lieberman 1985).

A reduction in presumed anxiety-inducing behaviors seems also to be a result of melatonin injection. In rats, for example, the administration of the indole decreases what is referred to as saccharin neophobia (Golus et al. 1979) while increasing exploratory behavior and decreasing postural freezing (Golus and King 1981).

Melatonin given by mouth in humans also changes the outcome of behavioral tests to which the individuals are subjected (Lieberman et al. 1984). In this study, three 80-mg doses of melatonin were given orally during a 2-hour period. Two hours before and 2 hours after melatonin treatment, each subject was asked to perform a battery of behavioral tests that measured aspects of performance, memory, and visual sensitivity and self-report mood questionnaires. The dosage of melatonin used in these studies was clearly pharmacologic, inasmuch as plasma levels of melatonin were roughly three orders of magnitude higher than normal daytime values in the treated subjects. As measured by the Profile of Mood States (McNair et al. 1971) and the Stanford Sleepiness Scale (Hoddes et al. 1973) (both self-report mood questionnaires), melatonin decreased alertness while increasing sleepiness (Lieberman et al. 1984), a change consistent with several published works. Melatonin also slowed choice reaction time but decreased errors of commission. Behavioral parameters that were not significantly influenced in this study included sustained fine motor performance and tests of memory and visual sensitivity. The conclusion was that melatonin has short-acting, sedative-like properties in humans. It is of interest, in fact, that the behavioral consequences of melatonin actually disappeared before plasma melatonin returned to daytime values.

Melatonin also seems to be involved in the synchronization of locomotor activity rhythms in animals and possibly also in humans; these effects would most likely be mediated by way of the central nervous system. Various studies in rats show that melatonin given on repeated days for a period of time synchronizes the free-running activity rhythms of the animals (Armstrong et al. 1986; Redman et al. 1983). This information stimulated investigations into the use of melatonin as a drug to treat jet lag, a phenomenon possibly related to the lack of synchrony of various rhythms to the circadian external environment. Preliminary results suggest that melatonin may have significant positive effects in overcoming the lethargy, confusion, and tiredness associated with jet lag (Arendt 1985). I can vouch for melatonin's efficacy as a jet-lag drug, having responded positively to its use during several trans-Atlantic trips in an easterly direction.

Besides melatonin, light has well-documented effects on the mood of humans (Kripke et al. 1984; Lewy and Sack 1986), and melatonin levels are reportedly "abnormal" in some depressed patients (Claustrat et al. 1984; Wetterberg et al. 1984). Whether, in fact, all of the effects of light in humans, e.g., on seasonal depression, relate to its ability to alter pineal melatonin synthesis or secretion remains uncertain (Terman et al. 1988; Wehr et al. 1986). The possible interactions of light, melatonin, and mood in humans will be reviewed in detail in subsequent chapters (see Chapters 3 and 5–7).

Endocrine and Psychoneuroendocrine Effects

The endocrine effects of the pineal gland and melatonin in experimental animals are now very well documented (Bittman 1984; Reiter 1980; Stetson and Watson-Whitmyre 1984). Whereas the bulk of these studies relate photoperiod and pineal physiology to reproductive function, all endocrine and perhaps most nonendocrine organs are influenced by the circadian production of melatonin by the pineal gland. In the final analysis, the pineal gland seems to function as an important annual synchronizer of organismal physiology. In the absence of this important time-keeping organ, either animals become aseasonal or their circannual rhythms are inappropriately timed.

In humans, a number of psychoneuroendocrine conditions may be directly or indirectly related to pineal function. In patients with anorexia nervosa, either no change (Brown et al. 1979; Dalery et al. 1985), a depression (Birau et al. 1984), or an elevation of nocturnal melatonin levels (Brambilla et al. 1988) has been reported. Although the results of these studies seem in conflict, several of the reports suffer from minimal statistical treatment of the data, and others examined only a small number of time points over a 24-hour period. Besides these findings, other workers also claim altered melatonin cycles in patients with either eating (Bolme et al. 1983; Tamarkin et al. 1982) or drinking (Borg et al. 1983) disorders or in patients with endocrine malfunctions (Berga et al. 1988; Fevre-Montange et al. 1983; Wetterberg 1978). From these studies, it is not possible to determine whether the reported changes in melatonin are either a cause or an effect of (or even clinically related to) the specific condition. Even if none of the conditions mentioned are related to the pineal gland and melatonin, surely disease states will be discovered that specifically relate to pineal malfunction. Like any other endocrine organ, the pineal must in some individuals function at either too high or too low a level; eventually these states would likely change the psychoneuro-endocrine state of the subject.

CONCLUSION

The pineal gland is a highly active organ of internal secretion in all animals, including humans. Its neural and endocrine consequences, as well as those of its chief secretory product, melatonin, are well documented in experimental animals. To deny an equally important role of the pineal gland and melatonin in humans would be naive and unwise. Certainly, an organ with such a high biosynthetic and secretory activity is not inconsequential in terms of human physiology.

REFERENCES

Antón-Tay F, Chou C, Anton S, et al: Brain serotonin concentration: elevation following intraperitoneal administration of melatonin. Science 162:277–278, 1968

Antón-Tay F, Diaz JL, Fernandez-Guardiola G: On the effect of melatonin upon the human brain: its possible therapeutic implications. Life Sci 10:846–850, 1971

Arendt J: Mammalian pineal rhythms, in Pineal Research Reviews, Vol 3. Edited by Reiter RJ. New York, Alan R Liss, 1985, pp 161–213

Arendt J, Wurz-Justice A, Bradtke J, et al: Long-term studies on immunoreactive human melatonin. Ann Clin Biochem 16:307–312, 1979

Armstrong SD, Cassone VM, Chesworth MJ, et al: Synchronization of mammalian circadian rhythms by melatonin. J Neural Transm [Suppl] 21:375–394, 1986

Berga SL, Mortola JF, Yen SSC: Amplification of nocturnal melatonin secretion in women with functional amenorrhea. J Clin Endocrinol Metab 66:242–244, 1988

Birau N, Alexander D, Bertholdt S, et al: Low nocturnal melatonin serum concentration in anorexia nervosa: further evidence for body weight influence. International Review of Clinical Science Medical Research 12:477–478, 1984

Bittman E: Melatonin and photoperiodic time measurement: evidence from rodents and ruminants, in The Pineal Gland. Edited by Reiter RJ. New York, Raven, 1984, pp 155–192

Bolme P, Hall K, Ritzen M, et al: Melatonin and cortisol secretion in children with Prader-Willi syndrome and with simple obesity. Neuroendocrinology Letters 5:408–413, 1983

Borg S, Mossber D, Wetterberg L: Low urinary melatonin concentration in alcoholics: a possible marker for a low central noradrenaline metabolism. Neuroendocrinology Letters 5:4–9, 1983

Brainard GC, Richardson BA, Petterborg LJ, et al: The effect of different light intensities on pineal melatonin content. Brain Res 233:75–81, 1982

Brainard GC, Richardson BA, King TS, et al: The influence of different light spectra on the suppression of pineal melatonin content in the Syrian hamster. Brain Res 294:333–339, 1984

Brainard GC, Lewy AJ, Menaker M, et al: Effect of light wavelength on the suppression of nocturnal plasma melatonin in normal volunteers. Ann NY Acad Sci 453:376–378, 1985

Brambilla F, Fraschini F, Esposti G, et al: Melatonin circadian rhythm in anorexia nervosa and obesity. Psychiatry Res 23:267–276, 1988

Brown GM, Kirwan P, Garfinkel P, et al: Overnight patterning of prolactin and melatonin in anorexia nervosa (abstract). Paper presented at the 2nd International Symposium on Clinical Psychoneuroendocrinology, Venice, Italy, 1979

Claustrat B, Chazot G, Brun J, et al: A chronobiological study of melatonin and cortisol secretion in depressed subjects: plasma melatonin, a biochemical marker in major depression. Biol Psychiatry 19:1215–1228, 1984

Craft CM, Morgan WW, Reiter RJ: 24-hour changes in catecholamine synthesis in the rat and hamster pineal glands. Neuroendocrinology 38:193–198, 1984

Cramer H, Rudolph J, Censbruch U, et al: On the effects of melatonin on sleep and behavior in man. Adv Biochem Psychopharmacol 11:187–191, 1974

Dalery J, Claustrat B, Brun J, et al: Plasma melatonin and cortisol levels in eight patients with anorexia nervosa. Neuroendocrinology Letters 7:164–169, 1985

Ebadi M: Regulation of the synthesis of melatonin and its significance to neuroendocrinology, in The Pineal Gland. Edited by Reiter RJ. New York, Raven, 1984, pp 1–37

Ebihara S, Marks T, Hudson HJ, et al: Genetic control of melatonin synthesis in the pineal gland of the mouse. Science 231:491–493, 1986

Fevre-Montange M, Tournaire J, Estour B, et al: Twenty four hour melatonin secretory pattern in Cushing's syndrome. Clin Endocrinol 18:175–182, 1983

Giarman NJ, Day M: Presence of biogenic amines in the bovine pineal body. Biochem Pharmacol 1:235–239, 1959

Golus P, King MG: The effects of melatonin on open field behavior. Pharmacol Biochem Behav 15:883–885, 1981

Golus P, McGee R, King MG: Attenuation of saccharin neophobia by melatonin. Pharmacol Biochem Behav 11:367–369, 1979

Gonzalez-Brito A, Jones DJ, Ademe RM, et al: Characterization and measurement of [125]iodopindolol binding in individual rat pineal glands: existence of a 24h rhythm in beta-adrenergic receptor density. Brain Res 438:108–114, 1988a

Gonzalez-Brito A, Reiter RJ, Menendez-Pelaez A, et al: Darkness-induced changes in noradrenergic input determine the 24 hour variation in beta-adrenergic receptor density in the rat pineal gland: in vivo physiological and pharmacological evidence. Life Sci 43:707–714, 1988b

Guerrero JM, Santana C, Reiter RJ: Protein synthesis, but not RNA transcription, is required for the isoproterenol induced activation of type-II 5′-deiodinase activity in the rat pineal gland. Neuroscience Research Communications 3:77–84, 1988

Hariharasubramanian N, Nair NPV, Pilapel C, et al: Plasma melatonin levels during the menstrual cycle: changes with age, in The Pineal Gland During Development. Edited by Gupta D, Reiter RJ. London, Croom-Helm, 1986, pp 166–173

Hedlund L, Lischko MM, Rollag MD, et al: Melatonin: daily cycle in plasma and cerebrospinal fluid of calves. Science 195:686–687, 1977

Hoddes E, Zarcone V, Smythe H, et al: Quantification of sleepiness: a new approach. Psychophysiology 10:431–436, 1973

Iguchi H, Kato KI, Ibayasaki H: Age-dependent reduction in serum melatonin concentrations in healthy human subjects. J Clin Endocrinol Metab 55:27–30, 1982

Illnerová H: Entrainment of mammalian circadian rhythms in melatonin production by light. Pineal Research Reviews 6:173–217, 1988

King TS, Steger RW, Steinlechner S, et al: Day-night differences in estimated rates of 5-hydroxytryptamine turnover in the rat pineal gland. Exp Brain Res 54:432–436, 1984a

King TS, Steinlechner S, Reiter RJ: Does maximal serotonin N-acetyltransferase activity necessarily reflect maximal melatonin production in the rat pineal gland? Neuroscience Letters 48:343–347, 1984b

Klein DC: Photoneural regulation of the mammalian pineal gland, in Photoperiodism, Melatonin and the Pineal. Edited by Reiter RJ. London, Pitman, 1985, pp 38–50

Klein DC, Weller JL: Indole metabolism in the pineal gland: a circadian rhythm in N-acetyltransferase. Science 169:1093–1095, 1970

Klein DC, Reiter RJ, Weller JL: Pineal N-acetyltransferase activity in blinded and anosmic rats. Endocrinology 89:1020–1023, 1971

Korf H-K, Møller M: The innervation of the mammalian pineal gland with special reference to central pinealopetal projection. Pineal Research Reviews 2:41–86, 1984

Kripke DF, Risch SC, Janowsky D: Bright white light alleviates depression. Psychiatry Res 10:105–112, 1984

Lewy AJ: Regulation of melatonin production in humans by bright artificial light: evidence for a clock-gate model and a phase response curve, in The Pineal Gland: Endocrine Aspects. Edited by Brown GM, Wainwright S. New York, Pergamon, 1985, pp 203–208

Lewy AJ, Newsome DA: Different types of melatonin circadian rhythms in some blind subjects. J Clin Endocrinol Metab 56:1103–1107, 1983

Lewy AJ, Sack RL: Light therapy and psychiatry. Proc Soc Exp Biol Med 183:11–18, 1986

Lewy AJ, Tetsuo M, Markey SP, et al: Pinealectomy abolishes plasma melatonin in the rat. J Clin Endocrinol Metab 50:204–207, 1980

Lieberman HR, Waldhauser F, Garfield G, et al: Effects of melatonin on human mood and performance. Brain Res 323:201–207, 1984

Matthews SA, Evans KL, Morgan WW, et al: Pineal indoleamine metabolism in the cotton rat, *Sigmodon hispidus*: studies on norepinephrine, serotonin, N-acetyltransferase and melatonin, in The Pineal and Its Hormones. Edited by Reiter RJ. New York, Alan R Liss, 1982, pp 35–44

McIntyre IM, Norman TR, Barrows GD, et al: Melatonin rhythm in plasma and saliva. J Pineal Res 1:177–183, 1987

McNair DM, Lorr M, Droppleman LF: Profile of Mood States Manual. San Diego, CA, Educational and Industrial Testing Service, 1971

Miles A, Philbrick DRS, Shaw DM, et al: Salivary melatonin estimation in clinical research. Clin Chem 31:2041–2042, 1985

Morgan RJ, Williams LM, Lawson W, et al: Stimulation of melatonin synthesis in ovine pineals in vitro. J Neurochem 50:75–81, 1988

Neuwelt EA, Lewy AJ: Disappearance of plasma melatonin after removal of a neoplastic pineal gland. N Engl J Med 308:1132–1134, 1983

Pang SF, Allen AE: Extra-pineal melatonin in the retina: its regulation and physiological function. Pineal Research Reviews 4:55–95, 1986

Pangerl B, Pangerl A, Reiter RJ, et al: Circadian variation of β-adrenoreceptor binding sites in the pineal gland of the Syrian hamster and prevention of the nocturnal reduction by light exposure or propranolol treatment. Neuroendocrinology 49:570–573, 1989

Pelham RW, Vaughan GM, Sandock KL, et al: Twenty-four-hour cycle of a melatonin-like substance in the plasma of human males. J Clin Endocrinol Metab 37:341–344, 1973

Perlow MJ, Reppert SM, Tamarkin L, et al: Photic regulation of the melatonin rhythms: monkey and man are not the same. Brain Res 180:211–216, 1980

Quay WB: Circadian rhythm in rat pineal serotonin and its modification by the estrous cycle and photoperiod. Gen Comp Endocrinol 3:473–479, 1963

Redman J, Armstrong S, Ng KT: Free-running activity rhythms in the rat: entrainment by melatonin. Science 219:1089–1091, 1983

Reiter RJ: Pineal interaction with the central nervous system. Waking Sleeping 1:253–258, 1977

Reiter RJ: The pineal and its hormones in the control of reproduction. Endocr Rev 1:109–131, 1980

Reiter RJ: Action spectra, dose-response relationships, and temporal aspects of light's effects on the pineal gland. Ann NY Acad Sci 453:215–230, 1985

Reiter RJ: Normal patterns of melatonin levels in the pineal gland and body fluids and experimental animals. J Neural Transm [Suppl] 21:35–44, 1986

Reiter RJ: The melatonin message: duration versus coincidence hypotheses. Life Sci 46:2119–2131, 1987a

Reiter RJ: Pineal-cerebrospinal fluid interactions. Wissenschaften Zeitschrift

Karl-Marx Universität Mathematic-Naturwissenschaften Reihe 36:35–39, 1987b

Reiter RJ: Pineal responses to stress: implications for reproductive physiology, in Biorhythms and Stress in Physiopathology of Reproduction. Edited by Pancheri P, Zichella L. New York, Hemisphere, 1988, pp 215–226

Reiter RJ, Sorrentino S Jr, Ralph CL, et al: Some evidence on the effects of blinding and anosmia in adult male rats with observations on pineal melatonin. Endocrinology 88:895–900, 1971

Reiter RJ, Hurlbut EC, Brainard GC, et al: Influence of light irradiance on hydroxyindole-*O*-methyltransferase activity, serotonin-*N*-acetyltransferase activity, and radioimmunoassayable melatonin levels in the pineal gland of the diurnally active Richardson's ground squirrel. Brain Res 288:151–157, 1983

Reiter RJ, Hurlbut EC, Esquifino AI, et al: Changes in serotonin levels in the pineal gland of the Richardson's ground squirrel in relation to the light-dark cycle. Neuroendocrinology 39:356–360, 1984

Reiter RJ, Esquifino AI, Champney TH, et al: Pineal melatonin production in relation to sexual development in the rat, in Pediatric Neuroendocrinology. Edited by Gupta D, Borrelli P, Attanasio A. London, Croom-Helm, 1985, pp 190–202

Reiter RJ, Joshi BN, Heinzeller TH, et al: A single 1 or 5 second light pulse at night inhibits hamster pineal melatonin. Endocrinology 118:1906–1909, 1986

Reiter RJ, Brit JH, Armstrong JD: Absence of a nocturnal rise in either NE, NAT, HIOMT or melatonin in the pineal gland of the domestic pig kept under natural environmental photoperiods. Neuroscience Letters 81:171–176, 1987a

Reiter RJ, Vaughan GM, Oaknin S, et al: Norepinephrine or isoproterenol stimulation of pineal *N*-acetyltransferase activity and melatonin content in the Syrian hamster is restricted to the second half of the daily dark phase. Neuroendocrinology 45:249–256, 1987b

Reppert SM, Perlow MJ, Klein DC: Cerebrospinal fluid metabolism, in Neurobiology of Cerebrospinal Fluid, Vol 2. Edited by Wood JH. New York, Plenum, 1980, pp 579–588

Reppert SM, Perlow MJ, Tamarkin L, et al: The effect of environmental lighting on the daily melatonin rhythm in primate cerebrospinal fluid. Brain Res 223:313–323, 1981

Rollag MD, Morgan RJ, Niswender GD: Route of melatonin secretion in the sheep. Endocrinology 102:1–8, 1978

Rollag MD, Panke ES, Trakulrungsi C, et al: Quantification of daily melatonin synthesis in the hamster pineal gland. Endocrinology 106:232–236, 1980

Rudeen PK, Reiter RJ, Vaughan MK: Pineal serotonin N-acetyltransferase in four mammalian species. Neuroscience Letters 1:225–229, 1975

Steinlechner S, Steger RW, King TS, et al: Diurnal variation in the serotonin content and turnover in the pineal gland of the Syrian hamster. Neuroscience Letters 35:167–172, 1983

Steinlechner S, Champney TH, Houston ML, et al: Simultaneous determination of N-acetyltransferase activity, hydroxyindole-O-methyltransferase activity and melatonin content in the pineal gland of the Syrian hamster. Proc Soc Exp Biol Med 175:93–97, 1984

Steinlechner S, King TS, Champney TH, et al: Pharmacological studies on the regulation of N-acetyltransferase activity and melatonin content of the pineal gland of the Syrian hamster. J Pineal Res 2:109–120, 1985

Steinlechner S, Stieglitz A, Heldmaier G, et al: Acute cold exposure reduces sensitivity of the Djungarian hamster pineal gland to light at night, in Abstracts of the 14th Congress of the European Society of Comparative Endocrinology. 1988, p 51

Stetson MH, Watson-Whitmyre M: Physiology of the pineal and its hormone melatonin in annual reproduction in rodents, in The Pineal Gland. Edited by Reiter RJ. New York, Raven, 1984, pp 109–154

Strada S, Klein DC, Weller J, et al: Effect of norepinephrine on the concentration of adenosine 3′,5′-monophosphate in rat pineal gland in organ culture. Endocrinology 90:1470–1475, 1972

Tamarkin L, Abastillas P, Chen HC, et al: The daily profile of plasma melatonin in obese and Prader-Willi syndrome children. J Clin Endocrinol Metab 55:491–496, 1982

Terman M, Terman JS, Quitkin FM, et al: Response of the melatonin cycle to phototherapy for seasonal affective disorders. J Neural Transm 72:147–165, 1988

Thiele G, Holtorf A, Steinlechner S, et al: The influence of light irradiance on pineal N-acetyltransferase activity and melatonin in the cotton rat, *Sigmodon hispidus*. Life Sci 33:1543–1547, 1983

Troiani ME, Reiter RJ, Tannenbaum MG, et al: Neither the pituitary gland nor the sympathetic nervous system is responsible for eliciting the large drop in elevated pineal melatonin levels due to swimming. J Neural Transm 74:149–160, 1988

Vacas MI, Lowenstein PR, Cardinali DP: Dihydroergocryptine binding sites in bovine and rat pineal glands. J Auton Nerv Syst 2:305–313, 1980

Vakkuri O: Diurnal rhythm in melatonin in human saliva. Acta Physiol Scand 124:409–412, 1985

Vanecek J, Sugden D, Weller J, et al: Atypical synergistic alpha$_1$- and beta$_1$-adrenergic regulation of adenosine $3',5'$-monophosphate in cultured rat pinealocytes. Endocrinology 116:2167–2173, 1985

Vaughan GM: Melatonin in humans, in Pineal Research Reviews, Vol 2. Edited by Reiter RJ. New York, Alan R Liss, 1984, pp 141–201

Vaughan GM, Reiter RJ: Pineal dependence of the Syrian hamster's nocturnal serum melatonin surge. J Pineal Res 3:9–14, 1986

Vaughan GM, Pelham PW, Pang SF, et al: Nocturnal elevation of plasma melatonin and urinary 5-hydroxyindoleacetic acid in young men: attempts at modification by brief changes in environmental lighting and sleep and by autonomic drugs. Endocrinology 42:752–764, 1976

Vaughan GM, Lasko J, Coggins SH, et al: Rhythmic melatonin response of the Syrian hamster pineal gland to norepinephrine in vitro and in vivo. J Pineal Res 3:235–250, 1986

Vollrath L, Semm P, Gammel G: Sleep induction by intranasal application of melatonin, in Melatonin—Current Studies and Perspectives. Edited by Birau N, Schloot W. London, Pergamon, 1975, pp 327–330

Waldhauser F, Steger G: Changes in melatonin secretion with age and pubescence. J Neural Transm [Suppl] 21:183–197, 1986

Webb SM, Champney TH, Lewinski AK, et al: Photoreceptor damage and eye pigmentation: influence on the sensitivity of rat pineal *N*-acetyltransferase activity and melatonin to light at night. Neuroendocrinology 40:205–207, 1985

Wehr TA, Jacobsen FM, Sack DA, et al: Phototherapy of seasonal affective disorder. Arch Gen Psychiatry 43:870–875, 1986

Weiss B, Strada BJ: Neuroendocrine control of the cyclic AMP system of brain and pineal gland. Adv Cyclic Nucleotide Res 1:357–374, 1972

Wetterberg L: Melatonin in humans: physiological and clinical studies. J Neural Transm [Suppl] 21:289–310, 1978

Wetterberg L: Clinical importance of melatonin. Prog Brain Res 52:539–547, 1979

Wetterberg L, Beck-Friis J, Kjellman BF, et al: Circadian rhythms in melatonin and cortisol secretion in depression, in Frontiers in Biochemical and Pharmacological Research in Depression. Edited by Usdin E. New York, Raven, 1984, pp 197–205

Wilkinson M, Arendt J, Bradtke J, et al: Determination of a dark-induced increase of pineal N-acetyltransferase activity and simultaneous radioimmunoassay of melatonin in pineal serum and pituitary tissue of the male rat. J Endocrinol 72:243–244, 1977

Wurtman RJ, Axelrod J: A 24-hour rhythm in the content of norepinephrine in the pineal gland and salivary glands of the rat. Life Sci 5:665–669, 1974

Wurtman RJ, Lieberman HR: Melatonin secretion as a mediator of circadian variations in sleep and sleepiness. J Pineal Res 2:301–303, 1985

Wurtman RJ, Axelrod J, Phillips LS: Melatonin synthesis in the pineal gland: control by light. Science 142:1071–1073, 1963

Zatz M: Pharmacology of the rat pineal gland, in The Pineal Gland, Vol 1. Edited by Reiter RJ. Boca Raton, FL, CRC Press, 1981, pp 229–242

Zatz M, Kebabian JW, Romero JA, et al: Pineal beta adrenergic receptor: correlation of binding of 3H-1-alprenolol with stimulation of adenylate cyclase. J Pharmacol Exp Ther 196:714–722, 1976

PART II

*The Pineal Gland and
Mood Disorders in Adults,
Adolescents, and Children*

Chapter 3

Melatonin as a Marker for a Subgroup of Depression in Adults

Lennart Wetterberg, M.D., Ph.D.
Johan Beck-Friis, M.D., Ph.D.
Bengt F. Kjellman, M.D., Ph.D.

Chapter 3

Melatonin as a Marker for a Subgroup of Depression in Adults

New diagnostic trends emphasize the importance of reliable biological markers to differentiate subtypes of depressive disorders. This differentiation will enable clinicians to choose the appropriate therapy for the individual patient and/or better predict the patient's response to different biological therapies such as pharmacotherapy, light therapy, or electroconvulsive therapy.

The basis for the interest in measuring melatonin in depressive disorders is related to, among others, a report by Wetterberg et al. (1979), in which one patient had higher cortisol levels during depression than during recovery, with a concomitant decrease in the nocturnal serum melatonin level from 0.12 nmol/L to 0.06 nmol/L. Also in this patient, the peak level of melatonin occurred earlier (midnight) during the depressive episode than during recovery (4 A.M.).

The potential use of melatonin as a biological marker in depression was obvious. Not only is melatonin dependent on both noradrenergic and serotonergic transmissions for its regulation (see Figure 3-1), it also seems to be related to the hypothalamic-pituitary-adrenal (HPA) axis (Figure 3-2), which is known to be affected in depressive states (elevated nocturnal cortisol levels and early escape in the dexamethasone suppression test [DST]).

Additionally, melatonin is useful in indicating the phase and the amplitude of the biological clock mechanism. The variation in melatonin concentrations over a 24-hour period allows scientists to study the hypothesis of free-running rhythm failure in subtypes of

This chapter was supported by grants from The Swedish Medical Research Council (3371), The Swedish Medical Society, Karolinska Institute, and St. Göran's Fund for Psychiatric Research.

depression and to test the phase-advance theory of affective illness introduced by Halberg (1968). Free-running rhythm refers to the genetically determined internal rhythm, which each healthy individual may display when isolated from all the external time cues. Normally, the internal body rhythm is synchronized with the external clock, i.e., the light-dark cycle arising from the sun-earth rotation. A free-running rhythm may be longer or shorter than 24 hours; this is the basis for the term *circadian*, meaning nearly 24 hours. *Phase advance* refers to a behavioral or hormonal rhythm with an appearance earlier than its normal circadian pattern.

The phase-advance theory of manic-depressive illness hypothesizes a pathological phase-advanced free-running rhythm, which is based on internal (e.g., body temperature rhythm versus sleep-wake cycle)

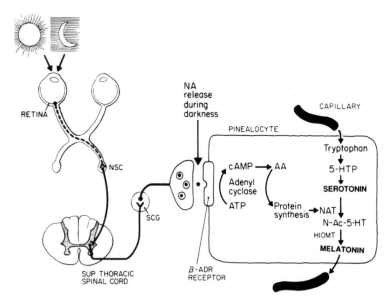

Figure 3-1. Melatonin rhythm-generating system (MRGS) includes eye, midbrain, and neuronal pathways to pineal gland. MRGS regulates conversion of serotonin to melatonin by noradrenergic receptor activity, which is influenced in a rhythmic fashion by variation in light-dark cycle and artificial light. AA, amino acids; HIOMT, hydroxyindole-*O*-methyltransferase; NA, noradrenalin; NAT, *N*-acetyltransferase; NSC, nuclei suprachiasmatici; SCG, superior cervical ganglia.

and external (e.g., body temperature rhythm versus light-dark cycle) desynchronization of physiological functions. The phase-advance theory was evaluated by Kripke (1983), who proposed that depression may be the result of an internal desynchronization of circadian oscillators, with the strong oscillator being phase advanced in relation to a weak oscillator. The internal rhythm could also be phase delayed, as has been proposed to be the case in seasonal affective disorder (SAD, "winter depression") (Lewy et al. 1987; Sack and Lewy 1988) (see Chapter 6).

Temporal external desynchronization such as in jet lag can occur in some individuals during flights over time zones. Rapid time-zone

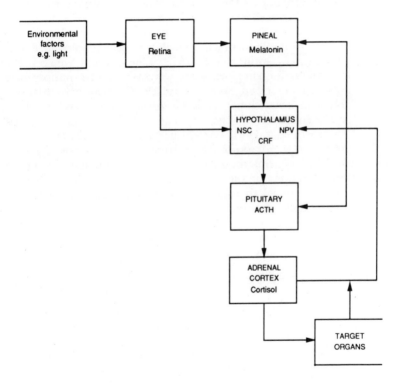

Figure 3-2.   Schematic model of hypothetical relationship between pineal gland and hypothalamic-pituitary-adrenal axis. NSC, nuclei suprachiasmatici; NPV, nuclei paraventricularis; CRF, corticotropin-releasing factor; ACTH, adrenocorticotropic hormone.

changes may even precipitate mood disorders in predisposed persons, as Jauhar and Weller (1982) showed in a study at Heathrow Airport in London.

Recently, Healy (1987) has convincingly argued for a "circadian rhythm dysfunction in affective disorders" linking "rhythm and blues" (p. 271). He claims that all mood disorders in some way involve a rhythm disturbance based on internal and/or external desynchronizations. It is obvious that as a rhythm-regulating factor and a marker for rhythm disturbances, melatonin offers a valuable tool in research on mood disorders.

MELATONIN AND SEASONAL VARIATION

Seasonal variations in the incidence of depression and suicide in mood disorders are well documented (Eastwood and Peacocke 1976; Eastwood and Stiasny 1978; Rosenthal et al. 1983). Circannual rhythms in pineal function in animals have been reported over the last two decades (Griffiths et al. 1979; Illnerová and Vanecek 1980). Seasonal variation in pineal gland weights in human autopsy material has been described (Wetterberg 1978). Seasonal variations in melatonin production measured in 24-hour serum levels and in urine have been shown at least on some latitudes (Arendt et al. 1977; Wetterberg et al. 1981; Wirz-Justice and Arendt 1979).

Based on these reports, it is probable that some forms of depression could be biochemically linked to a disturbance in melatonin production, secretion, or function. The close relationship between the pituitary, adrenal, thyroid, and gonadal systems and the pineal gland, and especially melatonin, may be reflected in corresponding neuro-psychoendocrine dysfunctions of clinical importance. Serum and plasma melatonin determinations may thus be of interest in relation to different disease states and diagnostic subgroups.

FACTORS INFLUENCING MELATONIN LEVELS IN SERUM

It is clear that factors other than psychiatric diagnoses are of importance for melatonin levels. It has been reported that bright light (Lewy et al. 1980; Wetterberg 1978), age (Attanasio et al. 1985; Iguchi et al. 1982; Nair et al. 1986; Sharma et al. 1989; Thomas and Miles 1989; Waldhauser and Waldhauser 1988, review; Wetterberg 1979), body weight (Arendt et al. 1982; Ferrier et al. 1982), body height (Beck-Friis et al. 1984), use of glasses (Erikson et al. 1983); use of drugs (e.g., β-adrenergic receptor blocking agents: Beck-Friis et al. 1983; Hanssen et al. 1977; Moore et al. 1979; chlorpromazine: Smith et al. 1979; antidepressant drugs: for review see Checkley and Palazidou 1988), and genetic variation (Wetterberg et al. 1983) are among factors that to different degrees and under various circumstances may influence melatonin levels in humans. Among these factors, age has been consistently connected with a concomitant reduction of melatonin levels. The influence of various drugs on melatonin metabolism is obvious, as well as the influence of possible differences in the assay methods used. (In our studies, the radioimmunoassay from KALAB [P.O. Box 634, Danville, CA 94526] for measuring melatonin in serum and urine has been used.)

In the evaluation of melatonin levels, after all of the above factors are considered, there is still support for a correlation between some subtypes of depression and melatonin concentrations.

MELATONIN IN DEPRESSION

In 1979, three research groups independently reported lowered nighttime melatonin concentrations in some depressed patients (Mendlewicz et al. 1979; Wetterberg et al. 1979; Wirz-Justice and Arendt 1979). In the same year, Lewy et al. (1979) reported an increase of melatonin levels during the manic phase compared with the depressive phase in one patient with a bipolar mood disorder. Wirz-Justice and Arendt (1979) found that hypomanic bipolar patients had the highest nocturnal melatonin levels, followed by depressed bipolar patients and after that depressed unipolar patients.

To follow up earlier findings of a possible relationship between the pineal gland and adrenal glands, Wetterberg et al. (1981) reported that low melatonin levels are related to high cortisol levels and an abnormal DST. The authors suggested that low melatonin levels in depression allowed for production of high levels of corticotropin-releasing factor (CRF). It seemed possible that melatonin or another pineal substance acted as a CRF-inhibiting factor under physiological conditions.

Several studies involving extensive neuroendocrine testing (e.g., of melatonin and cortisol secretion) have been reported over the past years (Table 3-1). As can be seen in Table 3-1, the association between low melatonin levels and certain types of depression or melancholia has been established in studies by several research groups. The association thus seems well documented. Three studies have not shown low melatonin in depressed patients (Jimerson et al. 1977; Stewart and Halbreich 1989; Thompson et al. 1988). Jimerson et al. used a bioassay, which has not been used in other studies. The patients were diagnosed as moderately to severely depressed, but no clinical

Table 3-1. Studies of melatonin levels in mood disorders

Reference	Assay	Diagnosis	Patients		Control subjects		Melatonin	HPA axis
			n(F)	Mean age (yr) (range)	n(F)	Mean age (yr) (range)		
Jimerson et al. 1977	Bioassay: urine	Depression; primary affective illness (RDC)	6(5)	33.7 (19–50)	6(2)	29.7 (19–65)	No change	
Wetterberg et al. 1979	RIA: serum	Depressive episode; remission; bipolar (RDC); rapid cycler	1(1)	48			Low in remission; decrease and phase advance in episode	Cortisol high in episode
Mendlewicz et al. 1979	RIA: plasma	Depressive episode: unipolar ($n = 3$), bipolar ($n = 1$)	4(4)	(37–61)	5(?)		No nocturnal rise in 3 patients	
Wirz-Justice and Arendt 1979	RIA: plasma	Depressive episode: unipolar ($n = 6$), bipolar ($n = 7$); hypomanic episode ($n = 5$)	13 depressive		5 hypomanic; 12 control		Morning levels significantly lower ($P < .001$) in unipolar depressive phase	
Lewy et al. 1979	Gas chromatography–mass spectrometry: plasma	Manic episode; bipolar	4		4		Significantly higher ($P < .01$) all day in manic episode	
Wetterberg et al. 1981	RIA: serum	Depressive episode; major depression (RDC)	12(7)	45 (27–62)			Patient with DST+ had lower melatonin	
Branchey et al. 1982	RIA: plasma	Depressive episode: unipolar ($n = 3$), bipolar ($n = 1$)	4(4)	47 (37–61)			Low (trait)	Cortisol high (state)

Reference	Method	Diagnosis	n	Age	n	Age	Findings
Beck-Friis et al. 1983, 1984, 1985a, 1985b	RIA: serum	Major depression (RDC); depressive episode (n = 32); recovery (n = 26)	32(18)	43 (26–63)	33(19)	40 (26–53)	DST+ associated with lowest melatonin	Negative regression: melatonin maximum at night; cortisol at 8 hours after dexamethasone administration 3 patients had DST+
Boyce 1985	Gas chromatography–mass spectrometry: urine	Melancholia (DSM-III)	8(7)	29 (22–25)			6-Sulfatoxy melatonin was not increased at night No clear association between melatonin and HPA axis
Steiner and Brown 1985	RIA: serum	Major depressive episode I (RDC)	25(16)	49 (21–82)			Low in I; lowest in II DST+ in 52% in I, 0% in II
		Personality disorder/superimposed depression II	8(4)	30 (21–57)			No association between low melatonin and DST+
Brown et al. 1985	RIA: serum	Melancholia (DSM-III) vs. control subjects	7(0)	42 (SE 4)	4(0)	32 (SE 5)	Lower in melancholia vs. nonmelancholia and controls
		Melancholia vs. non-melancholia vs. controls	19(14)	62.4 (SE 2.5)			No association between low melatonin and DST+
			9(9)	57.3 (SE 4.5)	7(0)	41.4 (SE 4.0) (19–65 in one elder, one younger group)	
Nair et al. 1984, 1985	RIA: plasma	Endogenous depression	9(5)	M 49.7, F 54 (43–67)	22(10)		Low in depression and aging High cortisol in depression

Table 3-1. Studies of melatonin levels in mood disorders (continued)

Reference	Assay	Diagnosis	Patients		Control subjects		Melatonin	HPA axis
			n(F)	Mean age (yr) (range)	n(F)	Mean age (yr) (range)		
Frazer et al. 1986		Major depression with melancholia (DSM-III) vs. controls	7(0)	42 (SE 4)	5(0)	32 (SE 5)	Lower in melancholia	
		Melancholia (DSM-III)	19(14)	62.5 (SE 2.5)			Lower in melancholia	
		Major depression without melancholia (DSM-III)	9(9)	57 (SE 4)	7(0)	41 (SE 4)	No association between low melatonin and DST+	
Brown et al. 1987	RIA: serum	Major depression (DSM-III)	28(23)	57 (SE 15)			Low in depression; correlates with depressed mood and reality disturbance	DST not shown
		Melancholia, nonmelancholia	19(14) melancholic, 9(9) nonmelancholic					

Almay et al. 1987	RIA: serum	Idiopathic pain syndrome (Williams and Spitzer 1982)	35(17)	44 (20–68)	53(28)	33.8 (20–63)	Low melatonin associated with depressive symptoms
Thompson et al. 1988	RIA: serum	Endogenous depression (RDC)	9(5)	48 (26–66)	9(5)	47 (28–58)	Paired controls showed no difference between depressed patients and controls
Kennedy et al. 1989	RIA: serum	Eating disorders (DSM-III-R)	33(33)	(18–40)			Patients with depressed status had significantly lower melatonin than patients with no depression and showed significantly lower melatonin-to-cortisol ratio
Stewart and Halbreich 1989	RIA: plasma	Major, minor intermittent depression (RDC)	113(52)	39.4 (18–63)			Elevation of daytime melatonin suggests nonspecificity of assay

Note. F, number of females in sample; HPA, hypothalamic-pituitary-adrenal; RDC, Research Diagnostic Criteria; RIA, radioimmunoassay; DST+, nonsuppression on dexamethasone suppression test.

ratings were shown. No difference was observed in the nocturnal melatonin rhythm between patients and control subjects during 1 or 2 baseline days, a sleep-deprivation day, and a recovery day. Although claiming the strength of matched control subjects in their study, the number of patients in the study by Thompson et al. is small ($n = 9$) and the matching of age, body height, and weight between patients and control subjects does not seem optimal according to the data presented. Furthermore, the selection and diagnoses of patients in this study seem mixed. Six patients were drug free for at least 1 year, and three were chronically depressed patients admitted for assessment for prefrontal lobotomy, who had been drug free for at least 6 weeks. Thus, the selection of the patients in this study differs from the selection of the patients in the Stockholm study (Beck-Friis 1983; Wetterberg et al. 1981). Patients with various mixtures of depression were included in the study by Stewart and Halbreich (1989). The authors mention that the high levels of daytime melatonin suggest a nonspecificity of the assay. In our opinion, these three studies do not convincingly refute the association between low melatonin and some types of depressive disorders.

Decreased melatonin secretion has also been found in childhood depression. Cavallo et al. (1987) studied 9 depressed boys (aged 7–13 years) and 10 control boys (aged 9–15 years) similar in pubertal development and found significantly lower mean 24-hour and mean overnight melatonin concentrations in the depressed patients (see Chapter 4).

The relation between low melatonin levels and disturbances in the HPA axis has been supported in many studies but not all and therefore needs further evaluation. Steiner and Brown (1985) and Brown et al. (1985) found melatonin levels to be decreased in depressed patients, but found no association between low melatonin levels and nonsuppression in the DST. Boyce (1985) found no clear association between melatonin secretion and the HPA axis. Lang and Sizonenko (1988) recently reviewed the literature on reported possible interactions between adrenal and pineal functions in mammals and found that no definite conclusions on this issue can be made as yet, but suggested a possible age-dependent relationship. Demisch et al. (1988) suggested in a study of dexamethasone administration in healthy subjects that dexamethasone affects nocturnal production of melatonin by means of mechanisms within the pineal gland. Kennedy et al. (1989) reported on melatonin and cortisol levels in 33 female patients with eating disorders compared with 10 female control subjects of comparable age. They found significantly higher nocturnal levels of plasma cortisol in the patients compared with the control subjects. Serum melatonin levels in the patients were initially similar to those of the control subjects; however, when patients were divided according to depression status, those with concurrent major depression had significantly lower nocturnal melatonin values than the nondepressed groups. The depressed patients in this study also had a significantly lower ratio of melatonin to cortisol. This ratio had earlier been proposed as a measure of the depressive state (Wetterberg et al. 1979, 1981). Current views on the use of melatonin as a tool in the diagnosis of mental disorders were reviewed in 1988 in the monograph *Melatonin: Clinical Perspectives* (Miles et al. 1988).

Specific findings relating serum melatonin to clinical variables in patients with depression have been reported by Wetterberg et al. (1981) and by Beck-Friis (1983) and Beck-Friis et al. (1984, 1985a, 1985b). The conclusions in these studies are based on the examination of 87 people, including acutely ill patients with major depression according to the Research Diagnostic Criteria (RDC) of Spitzer et al. (1978), patients in clinical remission, and healthy control subjects.

Brown et al. (1987), using the Hamilton factor scores (Rhoades and Overall 1983), reported correlation between clinical symptoms of depressed mood ($r = -.43$, $P < .04$), reality disturbance ($r = -.41$, $P < .04$), and melatonin, and a trend for correlation between sleep disturbance and melatonin ($r = -.33$, $P < .09$), but no correlation for symptom clusters of somatization, diurnal variation, agitation/anxiety, weight loss, or cognitive or vegetative factors. The symptom clusters of depressed mood also included motor retardation, inability to work, suicide items, indications of reality disturbance, symptoms of guilt feelings, depersonalization, and paranoid symptoms such as suspiciousness, referential thinking, and delusions.

In summary, nighttime melatonin levels may vary in different groups of depressed patients. Several studies have, however, found samples of patients with low nighttime levels of melatonin. We have studied the clinical features of such patients.

A LOW-MELATONIN SYNDROME IN DEPRESSION

The clinical finding of a subgroup of patients with low melatonin levels led us to study the possible existence of a "low-melatonin syndrome in depressed patients," which was introduced in 1983 (Beck-Friis 1983; Beck-Friis et al. 1985b). Our study included 32 acutely depressed inpatients diagnosed with major depressive illness according to RDC (Spitzer et al. 1978) and 33 healthy control subjects. Seventeen of the depressed patients had early escape of DST (serum cortisol not suppressed by dexamethasone) and 15 had a normal DST. Twenty-six of these patients were restudied 1 month to

1 year later while in a state of partial or complete remission. Clinical ratings were made with the Comprehensive Psychopathological Rating Scale (CPRS) (Åsberg et al. 1978). The study examined and in the statistical analysis adjusted background factors mentioned earlier in the section on melatonin in depression. We found that the depressed patients with early DST escape had significantly lower melatonin levels compared with depressed patients with a normal DST and the control group. The patients' use of drugs in the study did not influence the statistical outcome (Beck-Friis et al. 1984).

After adjustment for relevant influencing factors mentioned above, the results of our study (Beck-Friis et al. 1984, 1985a) showed no statistical difference in nocturnal maximum serum melatonin levels (MT_{max}) between the depressed patients (0.25 ± 0.03 nmol/L, mean $\pm$ SE) and the healthy control subjects (0.30 ± 0.03 nmol/L). However, when the depressed patients were divided into those with an abnormal response to the DST (DST+) and those with a normal response (DST−), a statistical difference was found. MT_{max} in the DST+ depressed patients ($n = 17$) was 0.19 ± 0.03 nmol/L and in the DST− group ($n = 15$) was 0.30 ± 0.03 nmol/L. The statistical analysis of the hypothesis of equal MT_{max} between the DST+, DST−, and control groups showed a significant difference in MT_{max} between the groups ($P = .004$).

Furthermore, a significant negative regression ($P = .04$) was found in the DST+ group between the MT_{max} level and the serum cortisol level at 8 A.M. after oral dexamethasone administration in those patients who did not suppress the cortisol below 200 nmol/L at 8 A.M. ($n = 8$). Their MT_{max} level was 0.17 ± 0.05 nmol/L, compared to 0.20 ± 0.02 nmol/L in those patients in the DST+ group who did suppress cortisol below 200 nmol/L at 8 A.M but not at 4 P.M. or 10 P.M. ($n = 9$).

When the depressed patients ($n = 26$) were restudied in clinical remission, the MT_{max} levels did not change significantly (0.24 ± 0.03 nmol/L in relapse; 0.23 ± 0.04 nmol/L in remission, NS). The same was true for the DST+ and DST− groups. In the DST+ group, the cortisol levels and the response in the DST normalized. This difference in melatonin and cortisol levels between relapse and remission led us to test the possibility of melatonin as a trait marker for certain types of depressions. Therefore, we further studied the clinical features of these patients (Beck-Friis et al. 1985b).

Patients with no reported diurnal variation of depressive symptoms ($n = 7$) had significantly lower MT_{max} levels (0.15 ± 0.05 nmol/L) than patients with reported diurnal variation ($n = 25$; 0.26 ± 0.03 nmol/L, $P = .047$). Patients with more than three registered depressive periods in the summer (June, July, and August) ($n = 12$) had significantly lower mean MT$_{max}$ levels (0.17 ± 0.04 nmol/L) than patients with three or less corresponding periods ($n = 20$). When the number of months with registered depressions was divided by the number of registered depressive episodes, patients in the DST+ group had a significantly higher quotient (7.4 ± 1.0 nmol/L) than patients in the DST− group (4.1 ± 0.2 nmol/L; $P = .01$), indicating that patients with abnormal DST have longer depressive episodes. A trend toward higher frequency of patients with more than three registered depressive periods during the summer was found in the DST+ group compared with the DST− group ($P = .08$). Eight of 12 (67%) of the patients in the DST− group but only 3 of 16 (19%) of the patients in the DST+ group reported an increase of depressive symptoms during the spring ($P = .02$). Patients in the DST+ group seemed to have their depressive episodes more equally distributed during the year, in contrast to the patients in the DST− group, who tended to have their depressive episodes more frequently in spring and autumn (Beck-Friis et al. 1985b).

These clinical findings in the depressed patients led us to the hypothesis of a "low-melatonin syndrome" in one subgroup of patients with depressive disorders. We therefore suggested that in these depressed patients, the following features constitute a low-melatonin syndrome: low nocturnal melatonin levels, an abnormal DST, a disturbed 24-hour rhythm of cortisol, and, as the main clinical feature, a less pronounced daily and annual cyclic variation in depressive symptomatology. Clinically, this means that the depression is more or less unlinked to the influence of external temporal cues. In this study, there was a correlation between low nocturnal melatonin levels and the symptoms of lassitude, sadness, and inability to feel, as reported on the CPRS clinical rating. Also, there was a correlation between low melatonin levels and a cluster of conative and emotional retardation symptoms. Findings by Brown et al. (1987) also support the correlation between low melatonin levels and depressed mood and/or retardation symptoms.

When looking at the relationship between low-melatonin syndrome and the diagnosis of melancholia in DSM-III (American Psychiatric Association 1980) and DSM-III-R (American Psychiatric Association 1987), the rigidity of the diagnostic criteria should be taken into consideration. Rigidity of the criteria may explain the lack of a correlation between low melatonin and melancholia in some studies. In DSM-III-R, the diagnosis of major depressive disorder with melancholic features is made by inclusion criteria such as early-morning awakening and symptoms worse in the morning. However,

Rafaelsen and Mellerup (1978) showed that the diurnal symptom variation disappeared during the most severe states of melancholia, but reappeared when the patients had started responding to treatment. Thus, the diurnal rhythm disturbances in melancholia are dynamic and not static.

Furthermore, in one Swedish study (von Knorring et al. 1977), early awakening and increased dysphoric mood in the early morning were not specific for "depressive syndrome" but were typically also seen in other diagnostic groups, e.g., anxiety disorders and neurotic depressions. Rhythmic variations of melancholic symptoms therefore seem to relate more closely to health than to the most severe state of melancholia.

In a chronobiological sense, health can be defined as the individual's maintained ability to make rhythms well functioning, i.e., to adapt external and internal biological rhythms. Melatonin and a normal pineal function seem to be involved in this adaptation. In depressed patients, low melatonin levels therefore hypothetically may impair this adaptation with a subsequent locked rhythmic capacity manifested in persistence of dysphoric mood and prolonged depressive episodes. The finding of our study that patients with low-melatonin syndrome could have longer depressive periods than patients with higher melatonin levels may also indicate that the low-melatonin patient group receives inadequate therapy.

Melatonin levels could serve as a marker for noradrenergic tone in the brain. If low melatonin concentrations reflect a deficiency of noradrenaline at receptor sites, the possibility that the low-melatonin syndrome might respond to noradrenergic antidepressive pharmacotherapy should be tested. A dysfunction in the serotonergic system could theoretically also lead to a low-melatonin syndrome.

On the functional level, low-melatonin syndrome in depression may be interpreted as a loss of rhythm amplitude, which could be a sign of dysfunction between the pineal gland and the suprachiasmatic nuclei in the hypothalamus. The findings by Reppert et al. (1988) of putative melatonin binding sites in the human "biological clock" (i.e., nuclei suprachiasmatici) are in line with such a hypothesis (see Figure 3-2).

The low nocturnal melatonin levels in these depressed patients could be genetically determined. Another or a parallel possibility is that the pineal and rhythmic function could be influenced by environmental factors in critical periods of life, e.g., impaired parent-child relationship, early psychic traumas, or other stressful factors in the first few years of life when the fundamentals of self-esteem and self-respect are laid down. Psychological injuries and traumas during such critical periods could hypothetically influence the ground for self-esteem according to the concepts of the narcissistic development formulated by Kohut (1971) and Kernberg (1975), and the soma, e.g., the endocrine system. Such a hypothesis is supported by the findings of Yuwiler (1985), who reported that steroid treatment in newborn rats reduces normal catecholamine-induced increase in pineal *N*-acetyltransferase (NAT) activity, indicating that stress in the neonatal period can alter pineal function. These animal studies support some of the psychoanalytic theories about the relationship between stress exposure and psychic trauma in early childhood and adult psychopathology. Breier et al. (1988) recently reported a significant correlation between early parental loss, development of adult psychopathology, and endocrine changes in the HPA axis with elevated levels of cortisol and adrenocorticotropic hormone (ACTH). In our above-mentioned study (Beck-Friis et al. 1985b), the depressed patients but not the healthy subjects who reported parental loss before age 17 had subnormal nocturnal melatonin levels and differed from patients with no reported parental loss.

The question arises whether low melatonin is a state or trait marker for depression (Miles and Thomas 1988; Sack and Lewy 1988). Relating melatonin and pineal function to the "rhythm-generating system" low melatonin in depressive states, as expressed in the low-melatonin syndrome, can be seen as a trait marker for the clinical time course of the depressive state. However, in other subtypes of mood disorders not related to low melatonin, e.g., in patients with bipolar disorders and hypothetically especially in "rapid cyclers" (i.e., patients with rapid and sudden mood swings), changes in the melatonin secretion amplitude may also be state dependent. This seemed to be the case in the first patient reported from our group (Wetterberg et al. 1979), who evidently was a "rapid cycler," and, although low in nighttime melatonin in the recovery state, her melatonin was further decreased during relapse. This also seems to be the case in patients responding to bright-light therapy.

EFFECTS OF 1-HOUR LIGHT EXPOSURE AND LIGHT THERAPY

Previous reports demonstrate that exposure of healthy persons to bright full-spectrum light with a luminance of 350 cd/m^2 (approximately 1500 lux) for 1 hour between 10 and 11 P.M causes a significant suppression of serum melatonin levels followed by a "rebound" of higher melatonin levels later in the night (Beck-Friis et al. 1985c; Beck-Friis et al. 1986). When the effects of 1-hour light exposure between 10 and 11 P.M. with three different luminances (50, 350, and 580 cd/m^2) were compared in eight healthy subjects, all three luminances significantly suppressed the melatonin secretion between 10 P.M. and midnight. However, only with a luminance of 350 cd/m^2 was a significant rebound effect found with increased melatonin secretion between 2 A.M. and 8 A.M. (Borg et al. 1987).

The same experimental paradigm was applied to 12 patients with a major depressive episode. In this group, the 1-hour light exposure of 350 cd/m^2 between 10 and 11 P.M. (light test) caused a significant acute suppression of the melatonin level, but there was no significant rebound as in healthy subjects (Kjellman et al. 1988).

Eight of the 12 depressed patients were treated with bright light according to the following plan. During the first night, blood samples were obtained with an indwelling catheter at 8 P.M., 10 P.M., 10:30 P.M., 11 P.M., midnight, 2 A.M., 4 A.M., 6 A.M., and 8 A.M. On the second night, sleep EEG was registered. On the 3rd day, a rating was done by two independent colleagues with the CPRS (Åsberg et al. 1978) and the Hamilton Rating Scale for Depression (Hamilton 1960). On the third night, blood samples were obtained as on the first night, with the exception that the patients were exposed to the light test. Light therapy was then given with indirect full-spectrum light exposure on 10 consecutive days between 6 and 8 P.M. with a luminance of 350 cd/m^2. The light therapy was given between November and March, when daylight ended before 6 P.M. After light therapy, the same investigative protocol was used as before therapy for three additional nights.

One aim of this study was to investigate the differences in melatonin rhythms before and after light therapy in patients who were responders or nonresponders to light therapy. Rigid criteria were used to determine responders: the patient had to be almost free of depressive symptoms and clinically recovered after 10 days of light therapy to be rated as a responder. With these criteria, five of eight patients were rated as responders.

Before light therapy, there was no significant rebound secretion of melatonin in these five patients (Figure 3-3). A tendency for phase delay of the melatonin curve and a narrower curve with a more distinct peak was seen after evening light therapy (Kjellman et al. 1988).

After light therapy, there was a clear reduction of melatonin secretion after the light test (Figure 3-4). The area under the curve was significantly reduced, and there was a phase delay of the secretion curve.

Thus, in the five patients who responded to light therapy, there was a tendency toward a phase delay and a narrower curve with a more distinct peak after evening light therapy. An increased sensitivity to the light test was also observed, resulting in a phase delay and significantly reduced melatonin secretion after light therapy. This increased sensitivity to evening light could be beneficial in depressed patients with phase advances of biological rhythms. The result could also be interpreted as an indication of a downregulation of β-adrenergic receptors, which can be seen in most antidepressant therapies.

Of the three nonresponders, two had no clear suppression of melatonin due to the light test. The third patient was the only one who showed subnormal melatonin levels before light therapy. After evening light, the melatonin secretion was abolished after the light test.

These results suggest that the clinical improvement of some depressed patients due to evening bright-light therapy may be related to an effect of bright light on "the melatonin rhythm-generating system." In the planning of light therapy, individual changes in

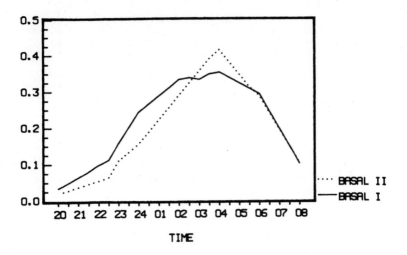

Figure 3-3. Nighttime serum melatonin (nmol/L) in five patients with depression responding favorably to bright-light therapy before (basal I) and after 10 days of 2-hour bright-light therapy of 350 cd/m^2 between 6 and 8 P.M. (basal II).

biological rhythms and individual sensitivity to light have to be taken into consideration.

These findings are in line with clinical observations of the low melatonin syndrome, in which normal pineal function is related to rhythmic functions of the pineal gland, whereas impaired pineal function is related to low melatonin levels and a loss of rhythmic functions of the pineal gland. Hypothetically, this loss may be responsible for the less favorable outcome of light therapy in patients with low-melatonin syndrome.

CONCLUSION

The secretion of melatonin is strongly influenced by environmental factors such as the light-dark cycle and also is dependent on neurotransmitter regulation of serotonin and noradrenaline. Chronobiological (circadian and circannual) aspects of mood disorders, such as mood swings and sleep problems, may also be related to

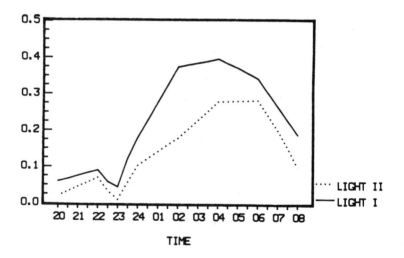

Figure 3-4.   Nighttime serum melatonin (nmol/L) during diagnostic light exposure for 1 hour between 10 and 11 P.M. in five patients with depression responding favorably to bright-light therapy. Light I, serum levels before light treatment. Light II, serum levels after 10 days of bright-light therapy of 350 cd/m² for 2 hours between 6 and 8 P.M.

disturbances in the function of the pineal gland and the secretion of melatonin. Measurement of melatonin is of potential clinical interest in diagnosing subgroups of mood disorders. Hitherto, measurements have been focused on depressive disorders because of the relative difficulties in doing laboratory research in patients in the manic phase of manic-depressive disorders.

Some patients with depressive disorders may exhibit the low-melatonin syndrome. In these patients, a diminished rhythmic functioning is manifested in the clinical symptoms as well as in endocrine parameters, i.e., the HPA axis. They also seem to have longer depressive phases. Identification of these patients may make it possible to provide more specific pharmacotherapy when the biochemical disturbances underlying this syndrome are better understood.

Patients with low-melatonin syndrome appear to differ clinically and biochemically from patients with depressive disorders with normal or high nocturnal melatonin levels, who seem to be more apt to relapse in a seasonal way. This latter group includes patients with SAD—"winter depression." Again, for this group, the use of the evening 1-hour light test described earlier may be a new tool for identifying responders to bright-light therapy. Hitherto, depressed patients with low-melatonin syndrome seemed to respond to a lesser degree to light therapy.

However, before melatonin levels can be used more generally in clinical practice for identification of depressive disorders, other factors influencing nocturnal melatonin secretion must be further understood and carefully considered.

In summary, melatonin levels in humans are influenced by genetic as well as environmental factors. The study of the pineal gland offers a natural pathway between the soma and the psyche for exploration of the chronobiological aspects of mood disorders.

REFERENCES

Almay B, von Knorring L, Wetterberg L: Melatonin in serum and urine in patients with idiopathic pain syndrome. Psychiatry Res 22:179–191, 1987

American Psychiatric Association: Diagnostic and Statistical Manual of Mental Disorders, 3rd Edition. Washington, DC, American Psychiatric Association, 1980

American Psychiatric Association: Diagnostic and Statistical Manual of Mental Disorders, 3rd Edition, Revised. Washington, DC, American Psychiatric Association, 1987

Arendt J, Wirz-Justice A, Bradtke J: Annual rhythm of serum melatonin in man. Neuroscience Letters 7:327–330, 1977

Arendt J, Hampton S, English J, et al: 24-hour profiles of melatonin, cortisol, insulin, C-peptide and GIP following a meal and subsequent fasting. Clin Endocrinol 16:89–95, 1982

Åsberg M, Montgomery SA, Perris C, et al: A comprehensive psychopathological rating scale. Acta Psychiatr Scand [Suppl] 271:5–27, 1978

Attanasio A, Borrelli P, Gupta D: Circadian rhythms in serum melatonin from infancy to adolescence. J Clin Endocrinol Metab 61:388–390, 1985

Beck-Friis J: Melatonin in depressive disorders—a methodological and clinical study of the pineal-hypothalamic-pituitary-adrenal cortex system. Unpublished academic thesis, Karolinska Institute, Stockholm, Sweden, 1983

Beck-Friis J, Hanssen T, Kjellman BF, et al: Serum melatonin and cortisol in human subjects after the administration of dexamethasone and propranolol. Psychopharmacol Bull 19:646–648, 1983

Beck-Friis J, von Rosen D, Kjellman BF, et al: Melatonin in relation to body measures, sex, age, season and the use of drugs in patients with major affective disorders and healthy subjects. Psychoneuroendocrinology 9:261–277, 1984

Beck-Friis J, Ljunggren JG, Thorén M, et al: Melatonin, cortisol and ACTH in patients with major depressive disorders and healthy humans with special reference to the outcome of the dexamethasone suppression test. Psychoneuroendocrinology 10:173–186, 1985a

Beck-Friis J, Kjellman BF, Aperia B, et al: Serum melatonin in relation to clinical variables in patients with major depressive disorders and a hypothesis of a low melatonin syndrome. Acta Psychiatr Scand 71:319–330, 1985b

Beck-Friis J, Borg G, Wetterberg L: Rebound increase of nocturnal melatonin levels following evening suppression by bright light exposure in healthy men: relationship to cortisol levels and morning exposure, in The Medical and Biological Effects of Light. Edited by Wurtman RJ. Ann NY Acad Sci 453:371–375, 1985c

Beck-Friis J, Borg G, Mellgren T, et al: Nocturnal serum melatonin levels following evening bright light exposure. Clin Neuropharmacol 9 (suppl 4):184–186, 1986

Borg G, Beck-Friis J, Kjellman BF, et al: Nocturnal serum melatonin levels in response to different intensities of evening bright light exposure in healthy man, in Fundamentals and Clinics in Pineal Research (Serono Symposia Publications, Vol 44). Edited by Trentini GP, De Gaetani C, Pévet P. New York, Raven, 1987, pp 361–364

Boyce PM: 6-Sulphatoxy melatonin in melancholia. Am J Psychiatry 142:125–127, 1985

Branchey L, Weinberg U, Branchey M, et al: Simultaneous study of 24-hour patterns of melatonin and cortisol secretion in depressed patients. Neuropsychobiology 8:225–232, 1982

Breier A, Kelsoe JR, Kirwin PD, et al: Early parental loss and development of adult psychopathology. Arch Gen Psychiatry 45:987–993, 1988

Brown RP, Kocsis JH, Caroff S, et al: Differences in nocturnal melatonin secretion between melancholic depressed patients and control subjects. Am J Psychiatry 142:811–816, 1985

Brown RP, Kocsis JH, Caroff S, et al: Depressed mood and reality disturbance correlate with decreased nocturnal melatonin in depressed patients. Acta Psychiatr Scand 76:272–275, 1987

Cavallo A, Holt K, Hejazi MS, et al: Melatonin circadian rhythm in childhood depression. J Am Acad Child Adolesc Psychiatry 26:395–399, 1987

Checkley SA, Palazidou E: Melatonin and antidepressant drugs: clinical pharmacology, in Melatonin: Clinical Perspectives. Edited by Miles A, Philbrick DRS, Thompson S. New York, Oxford University Press, 1988, pp 190–204

Demisch L, Demisch K, Nickelsen T: Influence of dexamethasone on nocturnal melatonin production in healthy adult subjects. J Pineal Res 5:317–322, 1988

Eastwood MR, Peacocke J: Seasonal pattern of suicide, depression and electroconvulsive therapy. Br J Psychiatry 129:472–475, 1976

Eastwood MR, Stiasny S: Psychiatric disorder, hospital admission and season. Arch Gen Psychiatry 35:769–771, 1978

Erikson C, Küller R, Wetterberg L: Nonvisual effects of light. Neuroendocrine Letters 5:412, 1983

Ferrier IN, Arendt J, Johnstone EC, et al: Reduced nocturnal melatonin secretion in chronic schizophrenia: relationship to body weight. Clin Endocrinol 17:181–187, 1982

Frazer A, Brown R, Kocsis J, et al: Patterns of melatonin rhythms in depression. J Neural Transm [Suppl] 21:269–290, 1986

Griffiths D, Seamark RFA, Bryden MM: Summer and winter cycles in plasma melatonin levels in the elephant seal. Aust J Biol Sci 32:581–586, 1979

Halberg F: Physiologic considerations underlying rhythmometry, with special reference to emotional illness. Paper presented at the Symposium Bel-Air III, Geneva, Masson et Cie, 1968, p 73

Hamilton M: A rating scale for depression. J Neurol Neurosurg Psychiatry 23:53–61, 1960

Hanssen T, Heyden T, Sundberg I, et al: Effect of propranolol on serum melatonin. Lancet 2:309, 1977

Healy D: Rhythm and blues: neurochemical, neuropharmacological and neuropsychological implications of a hypothesis of a circadian rhythm dysfunction in affective disorders (review). Psychopharmacology 93:271–285, 1987

Iguchi H, Kato KI, Ibayashi H: Age-dependent reduction in serum melatonin concentrations in healthy human subjects. J Clin Endocrinol Metab 55:27–29, 1982

Illnerová H, Vanecek J: Pineal rhythm in N-acetyltransferase activity in rats under different artificial photoperiods and natural daylight in the course of a year. Neuroendocrinology 31:321–326, 1980

Jauhar P, Weller MPI: Psychiatric morbidity and time zone changes: a study from Heathrow Airport. Br J Psychiatry 140:231–235, 1982

Jimerson DC, Lynch HJ, Post RM, et al: Urinary melatonin rhythms during sleep deprivation in depressed patients and normals. Life Sci 20:1501–1508, 1977

Kennedy SH, Garfinkel PE, Parienti V, et al: Changes in melatonin levels but not cortisol levels are associated with depression in patients with eating disorders. Arch Gen Psychiatry 46:73–78, 1989

Kernberg O: Borderline conditions and pathological narcissism. New York, Jason Aronson, 1975

Kjellman BF, Beck-Friis J, Borg G, et al: Nighttime melatonin in depressed patients: effects of one hour light exposure and light therapy (abstract). Psychopharmacology 96 (suppl):114, 1988

Kohut H: The Analysis of the Self. New York, International Universities Press, 1971

Kripke DF: Phase-advance theories for affective illness, in Circadian Rhythms in Psychiatry. Edited by Wehr TA, Goodwin FK. Pacific Grove, CA, Boxwood Press, 1983, pp 41–69

Lang U, Sizonenko PC: Melatonin and human adrenocortical function, in

Melatonin: Clinical Perspectives. Edited by Miles A, Philbrick DRS, Thompson C. New York, Oxford University Press, 1988, p 79–91

Lewy AJ, Wehr TA, Gold PW, et al: Plasma melatonin in manic-depressive illness, in Catecholamines: Basic and Clinical Frontiers, Vol 2. Edited by Usdin E, Kopin IJ, Barchas J. New York, Pergamon, 1979, pp 1173–1175

Lewy AJ, Wehr TA, Goodwin FK, et al: Light suppresses melatonin secretion in humans. Science 210:1267–1269, 1980

Lewy AJ, Sack RL, Miller S, et al: Antidepressant and circadian phase-shifting effects of light. Science 235:352–354, 1987

Mendlewicz J, Linkowski P, Branchey L, et al: Abnormal 24 hour pattern of melatonin secretion in depression. Lancet 2:1362, 1979

Miles A, Thomas DR: Melatonin and laboratory medicine, in Melatonin: Clinical Perspectives. Edited by Miles A, Philbrick DRS, Thompson C. New York, Oxford University Press, 1988, pp 253–279

Miles A, Philbrick DRS, Thompson C (eds): Melatonin: Clinical Perspectives. New York, Oxford University Press, 1988

Moore DC, Paunier L, Sizonenko PC: Effects of adrenergic stimulation and blockade on melatonin secretion in the human, in The Pineal Gland of the Vertebrates Including Man. Edited by Ariens Kappers J, Pevét P. Amsterdam, Elsevier North-Holland, 1979, pp 517–521

Nair NVP, Hariharasubramanian N, Pilapil C: Circadian rhythm of plasma melatonin in endogenous depression. Prog Neuropsychopharmacol Biol Psychiatry 8:715–718, 1984

Nair NVP, Hariharasubramanian N, Pilapil C: Circadian rhythm of plasma melatonin in endogenous depression, in The Pineal Gland: Endocrine Aspects (Advances in the Biosciences, Vol 53). Edited by Brown GM, Wainwright SD. Oxford, Pergamon, 1985, pp 339–345

Nair NVP, Hariharasubramanian N, Pilapil C, et al: Plasma melatonin—an index of brain aging in humans. Biol Psychiatry 21:141–150, 1986

Rafaelsen OJ, Mellerup ET: Circadian rhythms in depressive disorders, in Depressive Disorders. Stuttgart, FK Schattauer Verlag, 1978, pp 409–417

Reppert SM, Weaver DR, Rivkess SA, et al: Putative melatonin receptors in a human biological clock. Science 142:78–81, 1988

Rhoades HM, Overall JE: The Hamilton Depression Scale: factor scoring and profile classification. Psychopharmacol Bull 19:91–96, 1983

Rosenthal NE, Sack DA, Wehr TA: Seasonal variation in affective disorders, in Circadian Rhythms in Psychiatry. Edited by Wehr TA, Goodwin FK. Pacific Grove, CA, Boxwood Press, 1983, pp 185–201

Sack RL, Lewy AJ: Melatonin and major affective disorders, in Melatonin: Clinical Perspectives. Edited by Miles A, Philbrick DRS, Thompson C. New York, Oxford University Press, 1988, pp 205–227

Sharma M, Palacios-Bois J, Schwartz G, et al: Circadian rhythms of melatonin and cortisol in aging. Biol Psychiatry 25:305–319, 1989

Smith JA, Barnes JL, Mee TJ: The effect of neuroleptic drugs on serum and cerebrospinal fluid melatonin concentration in psychiatric subjects. J Pharm Pharmacol 31:246–248, 1979

Spitzer RL, Endicott J, Robins E: Research Diagnostic Criteria: rationale and reliability. Arch Gen Psychiatry 35:773–782, 1978

Steiner M, Brown GM: Melatonin-cortisol ratio and the dexamethasone suppression test in newly admitted psychiatry inpatients, in The Pineal Gland: Endocrine Aspects (Advances in the Biosciences, Vol 53). Edited by Brown GM, Wainwright SD. Oxford, Pergamon, 1985, pp 347–353

Stewart JW, Halbreich U: Plasma melatonin levels in depressed patients before and after treatment with antidepressant medication. Biol Psychiatry 25:33–38, 1989

Thomas DR, Miles A: Melatonin secretion and age (letter). Biol Psychiatry 25:364–367, 1989

Thompson C, Franey C, Arendt J, et al: A comparison of melatonin secretion in normal subjects and depressed patients. Br J Psychiatry 152:260–266, 1988

von Knorring L, Perris C, Strandman E: Diurnal variation in intensity of symptoms in patients of different diagnostic groups. Archiv Psychiatrie Nervenkrankheiten 224:295–312, 1977

Waldhauser F, Waldhauser M: Melatonin and aging, in Melatonin: Clinical Perspectives. Edited by Miles A, Philbrick DRS, Thompson C. New York, Oxford University Press, 1988, pp 174–189

Wetterberg L: Melatonin in humans: physiological and clinical studies. J Neural Transm [Suppl] 13:289–310, 1978

Wetterberg L: Clinical importance of melatonin. Prog Brain Res 52:539–547, 1979

Wetterberg L, Beck-Friis J, Aperia B, et al: Melatonin/cortisol ratio in depression. Lancet 2:1361, 1979

Wetterberg L, Aperia B, Beck-Friis J, et al: Pineal-hypothalamic-pituitary function in patients with depressive illness, in Steroid Hormone Regulation of the Brain. Edited by Fuxe K, Gustafsson JA, Wetterberg L. Oxford, Pergamon, 1981, pp 397–403

Wetterberg L, Iselius L, Lindsten J: Genetic regulation of melatonin excretion in urine. Clin Genet 24:403–406, 1983

Williams JBW, Spitzer JL: Idiopathic pain disorder: a critique of pain-prone disorder and a proposal for a revision of the DSM-III category psychogenic pain disorder. J Nerv Ment Dis 170:425, 1982

Wirz-Justice A, Arendt J: Diurnal, menstrual cycle and seasonal indole rhythms in man and their modification in affective disorders, in Biological Psychiatry Today. Edited by Obiols J, Ballús C, Gonzàles Monclús E, et al. Amsterdam, Elsevier North-Holland, 1979, pp 294–302

Yuwiler A: Neonatal steroid treatment reduces catecholamine-induced increases in pineal serotonin N-acetyltransferase activity. J Neurochem 44:1185–1193, 1985

Chapter 4

The Pineal Gland and Depressive Disorders in Children and Adolescents

Mohammad Shafii, M.D.
Michael B. Foster, M.D.
Richard Greenberg, Ph.D.
Ann McCue Derrick, R.N., M.S.
Mary P. Key, M.S., M.T.(ASCP)

Chapter 4

The Pineal Gland and Depressive Disorders in Children and Adolescents

PSYCHOBIOLOGY OF DEPRESSION IN CHILDREN AND ADOLESCENTS

During the last 10–15 years, investigators have begun exploring the psychological factors contributing to or correlating with the development of depressive disorders and suicidal behavior in children and adolescents (Carlson and Cantwell 1982; Kashani et al. 1981; Kovacs and Beck 1977; Poznanski et al. 1979, 1984; Puig-Antich 1980; Shafii and Shafii 1982a, 1982b). Based on these studies, depressive disorders in children and adolescents are now viewed as similar to those in adults, and the same criteria are used for diagnosis (DSM-III and DSM-III-R [American Psychiatric Association 1980, 1987]).

Few researchers have studied the biological factors contributing to depressive disorders in children and adolescents. Cytryn et al. (1974) measured levels of norepinephrine in the urine of chronically depressed children versus a normal control group and found that the level of norepinephrine was lower in six of eight depressed patients. Also, deviations in the level of 3-methoxy-4-hydroxyphenylethyl glycol (MHPG), a metabolite of norepinephrine, were found as compared with control subjects, "although no consistent directional pattern was apparent" (Cytryn et al. 1974, p. 660). Later, McKnew and Cytryn (1979) found that MHPG was higher in the urine of depressed children than in the urine of the control group.

We wish to thank S.L. Shafii for her significant editorial contribution and J. Steltz-Lenarsky and G. Kaller for their help as research and program assistants. We also are grateful to D.R. MacMillan, Department of Pediatrics, University of Louisville School of Medicine, and L. Wetterberg, Karolinska Institute, Stockholm, Sweden, for the use of their laboratories.

Dexamethasone Suppression Test

In recent years, the dexamethasone suppression test (DST) has been used as a possible biological marker for melancholic depression in adults (Carroll 1982a, 1982b; Carroll et al. 1968, 1976, 1981) and also in children and adolescents (Crumley et al. 1982; Extein et al. 1982; Geller et al. 1983; Ha et al. 1984; Hsu et al. 1983; Livingston et al. 1984; Poznanski et al. 1982; Robbins et al. 1982, 1983; Weller et al. 1984). Approximately 30–60% of adult patients suffering from melancholic depression have early escape of dexamethasone (Carroll et al. 1981; Meltzer and Fang 1983). Similar results have been reported from studies involving children and adolescents (Khan 1987; Klee and Garfinkle 1984). Other studies show that early escape is not only related to melancholic depression but may also be related to alcoholism, weight loss, anxiety disorder, and other illnesses such as bulimia and diabetes mellitus (Feinberg and Carroll 1984; Hudson et al. 1982, 1984; Swartz and Dunner 1982). In these studies, dexamethasone is seen as a biological marker reflecting the physical or emotional *state* of the individual, rather than as an indicator of the biological *trait* of depression.

Growth Hormone and Major Depression

Puig-Antich et al. (1984a, 1984b) measured baseline growth hormone, cortisol, and prolactin levels in the serum of prepubertal children, ages 6–12. Thirteen of these children suffered from endogenous major depression according to Research Diagnostic Criteria (RDC) (Feighner et al. 1972). The RDC describe endogenous major depression as a subtype of major depression in which a patient shows a distinct quality of sadness (a feeling different from that following the death of a loved one), lack of reactivity to the environment, and worse mood in the morning. At the same time, the patient must meet the following RDC criteria for major depression: 1) dysphoric mood or pervasive loss of interest or pleasure lasting 2 weeks and resulting in impairment of functioning or requiring treatment; 2) five of eight symptoms (increased or decreased appetite or weight loss or gain, increase or decrease in sleep, fatigue or loss of energy, psychomotor agitation or retardation, loss of interest or pleasure in usual activities, feeling of self-reproach or inappropriate guilt, diminished ability to think or concentrate, and suicidal ideation, threats, or attempts); and 3) no symptoms of schizophrenia (Robins et al. 1982; Spitzer et al. 1978).

The investigators (Puig-Antich et al. 1984a) performed an insulin tolerance test (ITT) by injecting the subjects with insulin (0.1 U/kg body weight). The children with endogenous depressive disorder had significant hyposecretion of growth hormone in response to insulin, compared with both the children with nonendogenous depressive disorder and the nondepressed neurotic children. Baseline and post-ITT levels of prolactin and cortisol did not differ among the three subgroups during a depressive episode.

Puig-Antich et al. (1984c) also studied the response to insulin in 18 prepubertal children after at least a 4-month recovery from a depressive disorder. In this group, 11 had endogenous depression, 7 had nonendogenous depression, and 16 had neurotic disorders other than depression. Children with past endogenous depression continued to have significant hyposecretion of growth hormone compared with the other groups. The investigators concluded that "a [growth hormone] hyporesponse to ITT may be a true marker of a past episode or of trait for endogenous major depressive disorder in prepuberty" (p. 471).

THE PINEAL GLAND AND MELATONIN

It is only within the last 30 years that we have begun to understand the functions of the pineal gland. In 1958, Lerner et al. (1958, 1959) identified the pineal indole hormone melatonin (N-acetyl-5-methoxytryptamine). Shortly thereafter, Axelrod and Weissbach (1960) showed that melatonin was a metabolite of serotonin and described its biosynthesis as taking place in the pineal gland. Wurtman et al. (1964) described melatonin as a biological marker for the pineal gland and conducted studies on the effect of light on melatonin synthesis. These investigators have shown that melatonin production is stimulated by darkness and inhibited by light (see Chapters 1 and 2).

Anton-Tay et al. (1971) observed that a single dose of melatonin (1.25 mg/kg body weight) administered to normal subjects created temporary sleepiness and "a sensation of well-being, and moderate elation" (p. 843). Cramer et al. (1974) noted that 50 mg of melatonin administered to normal subjects cut the onset of sleep in half as compared with a control group. On the other hand, Carmen et al. (1976) reported a significant contrast after administering melatonin to six moderately to severely depressed patients. Symptoms of depression increased, and patients suffered weight and appetite loss and a drop in oral temperature.

Arendt et al. (1975) and Wetterberg et al. (1978), among others, developed a method of radioimmunoassay for the direct measurement of melatonin in the pineal gland and in body fluids such as urine, blood, and cerebrospinal fluid. Although melatonin excretion is fairly consistent for an individual from day to day, seasonal variations in morning (postpeak) melatonin levels have been reported (Beck-Friis et al. 1984; Zetin et al. 1987).

The Pineal Gland and Puberty

The physiological role of the pineal gland is still not well understood. However, animal studies suggest that it may play a major role in the reproductive process (Johnson and Reiter 1978; Reiter 1968; Shivers and Yochim 1979; Tamarkin et al. 1976, 1985). Kitay (1954) found an association between hypoactive pineal tumors and precocious puberty and also an association between hyperactive tumors and delayed puberty in males. Silman et al. (1979) measured daytime serum levels of melatonin, luteinizing hormone, follicle-stimulating hormone, testosterone, and estradiol in 51 healthy boys and girls between the ages of 11.5 and 14 years in the United Kingdom. They found a highly significant drop in the serum concentration of melatonin with advancing development in the boys. There was no difference in the melatonin levels of the girls at different stages of development. The authors hypothesized that "it is possible that the drop in melatonin, which we have observed, is part of the process which initiates the physical and endocrine changes of puberty" (Silman et al. 1979, p. 302). In addition, they stated that the lack of change in the melatonin level in the girls "may indicate that there is a sex difference in pineal endocrinology" (p. 302). Beck-Friis et al. (1984) reported higher melatonin levels in females than in males; however, they suggested that the difference was not significant when adjusted for height. An overall significant negative correlation was found between body weight and serum melatonin levels; that is, lower melatonin values were found in taller and/or heavier persons. Recent thinking attributes the decrease of melatonin in adolescent males to the increase of body weight rather than to sex differences (see Chapter 5).

Lenko et al. (1982), on the other hand, found no significant differences between daytime plasma melatonin levels of males and females in different pubertal stages and concluded that "the onset of puberty is not associated with changes in melatonin secretion, as estimated from plasma melatonin levels" (p. 1056). They noted that daytime plasma samples may not be ideal for studying melatonin levels because "important changes in total daily melatonin secretion may remain unnoticed when determining only daytime melatonin levels" (p. 1057). Melatonin secretion follows a constant circadian rhythm, peaking in the plasma, cerebrospinal fluid, and urine between 11 P.M. and 2 A.M. (Lynch et al. 1975).

Melatonin and Depressive Disorders in Adults

Beck-Friis et al. (1984), in Stockholm, Sweden, studied serum melatonin levels in 30 patients with major depressive disorders, 24 patients in remission from unipolar and bipolar major affective disorders, and 33 healthy control subjects (see Chapter 3). They found that peak melatonin levels were lower in both patient groups compared with the control group. In another portion of the study, the seasonal variation of plasma melatonin was investigated in two groups: one group with 19 individuals who were studied from November to January during the winter or "dark period" and the other group with 31 individuals who were studied from April to July during the spring-summer or "bright period." Significantly lower levels of melatonin were found in samples obtained during the bright period (postpeak). They concluded that the seasonal difference in postpeak levels may reflect "a suppression of melatonin by the bright light of the morning" (Beck-Friis et al. 1984, p. 274).

Lewy et al. (1980, 1982, 1987) and Rosenthal et al. (1984, 1985) conducted studies at the National Institutes of Health on a type of depression known as seasonal affective disorder (SAD), which appears to be triggered by a decrease in day length as winter approaches. Lewy et al. (1980) determined that bright artificial light—at least 10 times brighter than ordinary room light—suppresses melatonin secretion in humans (see Chapter 6).

Rosenthal et al. (1984) reported on a study of 29 patients with a history of mood disorder who had experienced at "least two consecutive years in which depression had developed during the fall or winter and remitted during the following spring or summer" (p. 72). Most of the depressive episodes began in October, November, or December and ended in March. In addition, 66% (19) of these patients reported that their depression was alleviated when they traveled south and intensified when they traveled north.

In the study by Rosenthal et al., light treatment was administered to 11 of 18 patients who had become "moderately depressed" for at least 2 weeks as determined by clinical judgment and substantiated by scores on the Hamilton Rating Scale for Depression (Hamilton 1960, 1976) and the Beck Depression Inventory (Beck and Beamesderfer 1974; Beck et al. 1961). Patients were randomly assigned to sit in front of either bright white fluorescent light (approximately 2,500 lux) or dim yellow fluorescent light (approximately 100 lux) in their homes for 3 hours after dawn and 3 hours after dusk. The patients were evaluated after 2 weeks. They found that bright white light had a significant therapeutic effect in patients suffering from SAD. These findings were further reported in a subsequent crossover study (Rosenthal et al. 1985). Rosenthal suggests that bright-light therapy may be effective in the treatment of SAD "due to the suppressant effect of bright light on the pineal hormone melatonin" (p. 169).

Wetterberg and his colleagues at the Karolinska Institute in Stockholm, Sweden, have conducted numerous studies both on the relationship between circadian rhythm and the secretion of melatonin and on the relationship between melatonin and depressive disorders (Wetterberg 1978, 1983; Wetterberg et al. 1978, 1984). Wetterberg (1983) studied 32 patients with "acute major depressive disorder." He divided the patients into two groups: 1) 17 with an abnormal DST (early escape) and 2) 15 with a normal DST. He noticed that the patients with early escape of cortisol had lower serum melatonin levels than patients with a normal DST. He also noticed that, even after recovery from a depressive episode, the patients with early escape and low melatonin levels still had lower levels of melatonin than the other group. They concluded that lower levels of serum melatonin in depressed patients with early escape from DST are a biological *trait* marker for depression (see Chapter 3).

Melatonin and Depressive Disorders in Children and Adolescents

Cavallo et al. (1987) have published the only study that we were able to find regarding melatonin levels in depressed children and adolescents. They reported on the mean of integrated plasma melatonin of 9 children and adolescents aged 7–13 years and 10 control subjects aged 9–15 years. Based on DSM-III criteria, 4 children from the experimental group were diagnosed with major depression, 4 with atypical depression, and 1 with dysthymic disorder. The mean nighttime melatonin level in depressed patients was 50.7 pg/ml (SD 17.8), compared to 75.7 pg/ml (±20.0) in the control group ($P <$ .05). They concluded that "melatonin secretion is decreased in childhood depression" and that there were "no differences between melatonin concentration of children with major depression and those with other forms of depression" (p. 398).

The study by Cavallo et al. has major methodological problems: 1) The number of experimental and control subjects is small. 2) Various depressive disorders are mixed together. Four of the nine patients are referred to as "atypical depression," which is not defined. According to DSM-III, atypical depression is a "residual category for individuals with depressive symptoms who cannot be diagnosed as major depressive, dysthymic, or adjustment disorders" (p. 223). 3) Patients' secondary diagnosis(es), which may make the research group less homogeneous, have not been taken into consideration.

A STUDY OF BEDTIME AND OVERNIGHT URINARY MELATONIN

To explore whether a relationship exists between melatonin levels and depressive disorders in children and adolescents, we measured melatonin levels in bedtime and overnight urine samples of patients admitted to an inpatient child psychiatric setting at the University of Louisville School of Medicine, Louisville, Kentucky.

Research Setting

The inpatient child psychiatric service is an acute short-term pediatric-psychiatric unit located in Kosair Children's Hospital, Louisville, Kentucky. This 227-bed acute-care children's hospital is a service, teaching, and research center for the Department of Pediatrics and Child Psychiatric Services of the University of Louisville School of Medicine. Children and adolescents ages 2–16 years are admitted to this inpatient service. The average stay is 14–21 days. The patients are usually on a regular diet and follow similar schedules and activities. The younger patients go to bed at 9 P.M., and the older ones between 9:30 and 10 P.M. Lights are off in the patients' bedrooms when they are sleeping. Patients usually arise between 6:30 and 7:30 A.M. Each semiprivate bedroom area, which accommodates two to four children, has a bathroom (Shafii et al. 1979).

Methods

Children and adolescents ages 6–16 years admitted to the inpatient child psychiatric service were asked to participate in this study, which was approved by the University of Louisville Medical School Human Studies Committee. Informed consent was obtained from patients and their parent(s) or guardian(s).

Each patient was interviewed separately by the senior investigator, a child psychiatrist (M.S.), and by an experienced child psychiatric nurse clinical specialist (A.M.D.). During the structured interviews, the following instruments were administered to assess the presence or absence of depression:

1. *Children's Depression Inventory (CDI).* The CDI (Kovacs 1981; Kovacs and Beck 1977) is a 27-item, self-report, symptom-oriented scale designed for children ages 8–13 years, but is suitable

for children as young as 6 years (first-grade reading level) and as old as 17 years. It is modeled after the Beck Depression Inventory (Beck et al. 1961) for adults and was the first self-report measure used in childhood depression research. Each item of the inventory relates to overt symptoms of depression such as sadness or sleep or appetite disturbance. Given three sentences indicating varying severity for each item, the child must choose the one that best describes him or her for the past 2 weeks. An interviewer can read aloud each item with the child or allow older subjects without reading difficulties to complete the inventory on their own. In this study, an investigator read each item aloud to the patient. A CDI score of 19 or more is suggestive of depression.

2. *Children's Depression Rating Scale—Revised (CDRS-R)*. The CDRS (Poznanski et al. 1979, 1984) is a clinician-rated scale for the assessment of depression in children ages 6–12 years. A revised version, the CDRS-R, incorporates changes made in the instrument since its inception. The CDRS-R has 17 items, including questions on such symptoms as pathological guilt, tempo of speech, suicidal ideation, and fatigue. The clinician rates the child's answers on a 7-point severity scale. Out of a possible total of 113 points, a CDRS-R score of 40 or more usually indicates a clinical depression. We found that the CDRS-R was also useful for adolescents ages 13–16 years.

3. *Child Behavior Checklist (CBCL) and Youth Self-Report (YSR)*. The CBCL is a 120-item, parent or guardian report designed to score the social competence and behavior problems of children ages 4–16 years. The CBCL can be self-administered or read by an interviewer and is then scored on the basis of the normed Child Behavior Profile (Achenbach 1978; Achenbach and Edelbrock 1979). The investigators in this study read aloud each item of the YSR to the patients.

4. *Hopelessness Scale (HS)*. Beck (1978) developed a 20-item, true-false questionnaire for adults and adolescents ages 13 years and older that elicits the degree of pessimism and hopelessness. We used Beck's HS for adolescents ages 13 years and older.

5. *Hopelessness Scale for Children*. To assess the degree of hopelessness in children ages 6–13 years, Kazdin et al. (1986) modified Beck's HS and developed a 17-item, true-false questionnaire to assess hopelessness in this age-group. We used this scale for children ages 6–13 years.

6. *Anthropometric and pubertal staging data—Tanner's stages*. Patients' height and weight were measured, and they were evaluated for stages of pubertal development according to Tanner

(1962) by one of the investigators, a pediatric endocrinologist (M.B.F.) Anthropometric data were used to estimate the body surface area of each subject. Historical information regarding age at menarche and date of most recent menstrual period were obtained from female subjects.

7. In addition to the administration of the above instruments for research purposes, patients' hospital records, particularly psychiatric and pediatric admission notes, psychological testing results, electroencephalogram, complete blood count, urinalysis, other laboratory findings, and the discharge summary, were reviewed.

Biological Data

Due to the circadian rhythm of melatonin, continuous blood sampling through catheters is probably the most accurate method of determining melatonin levels. However, considering numerous factors, including the age of the subjects, we decided to use a nonintrusive sampling method. The highest serum melatonin level is reached between 11 P.M and 3 A.M., with a peak around 2 A.M. (Wetterberg et al. 1978). Wetterberg (1978) reported that there is a correlation ($r = .89$) between serum melatonin level at 2 A.M. and urinary melatonin level on morning awakening. Overnight urine collection is an effective and nonintrusive method for obtaining melatonin levels.

During the patients' hospitalization, two to three pairs of bedtime and overnight urinary samples were collected and stored on ice. The samples were coded to ensure blindness and submitted for assay to the laboratory. Aliquots from coded samples were stored frozen until final preparation for the radioimmunoassay and remained blinded with respect to time of collection and source. Urinary melatonin levels were measured with a single-antibody radioimmunoassay (Wetterberg et al. 1978), which uses a rabbit antiserum, a melatonin standard (KALAB, Danville, California), and a tritiated melatonin tracer (New England Nuclear, Boston, Massachusetts).

Results

DSM-III diagnostic criteria for major depressive disorder, dysthymic disorder, conduct disorder, oppositional disorder, adjustment disorder, and others were arranged in a checklist (Shafii et al. 1988). Psychiatric, psychological, and developmental research data along with the patients' hospital records were reviewed, and relevant DSM-III criteria were checked off independently by two members of the research team (M.S. and A.M.D.). Then the two researchers discussed their observations and impressions and determined a research diagnosis(es) by consensus.

Based on the research diagnosis(es), 96 patients were divided into three groups:

1. *Group I*—primary depression: major depression, major depression superimposed on dysthymic disorder, or dysthymic disorder ($N = 21$). Because these patients did not have any other psychiatric disorder in the past or at the present time, they were diagnosed as having primary depression.
2. *Group II*—secondary depression: major depression/dysthymic disorder associated with anxiety disorder, conduct disorder, or psychotic or identity disorder; adjustment disorder with depressed mood and mixed disturbances of emotion and conduct ($N = 36$). In this group, depressive disorders were associated with other psychiatric disorders and thus patients were diagnosed as having secondary depression.
3. *Group III*—control group: conduct disorder and/or oppositional disorder in some cases associated with attention-deficit disorder with hyperactivity ($N = 39$).

Data were analyzed by Minitab Data Analysis Software (1985). Multiple regression analysis was used to perform the covariate analyses.

Demographic and developmental data. Of the 96 patients, 56% were male and 44% female; 62% were white and 38% black; and 33% were children ages 6–11 years and 67% adolescents ages 12–16 years. Regarding stages of pubescence, 39% were in Tanner stages 1 and 2 and 61% were in Tanner stages 3–5.

Overnight urinary melatonin. The overnight urine specimen included any urine voided after the patient went to bed and the first voided specimen on awakening in the morning. The mean of 2 or 3 overnight urinary melatonin samples in Group I was significantly higher than in the other two groups: Group I, 0.438 ± 0.031 (SD = 0.147) nmol/L; Group II, 0.275 ± 0.024 (SD = 0.121) nmol/L; and Group III, 0.273 ± 0.023 (SD = 0.156) nmol/L; $P < .001$. Multiple comparison tests based on Scheffé's (1959) method showed Group I to be significantly different from Groups II and III. After simultaneous adjustment for age, sex, race, height, and weight, the mean of overnight urinary melatonin in Group I remained significantly higher than in the other two groups ($P < .01$). Also, adjustment for Tanner stages and the season of the year had no effect.

As mentioned earlier, Wetterberg et al. (1984), in depressed adults with early escape of dexamethasone, and Cavallo et al. (1987), in depressed children and adolescents, found a decrease of serum melatonin. In contrast, we found a significant increase of overnight urinary melatonin in primary depression compared with secondary depression or conduct and/or oppositional disorders.

SUMMARY AND DISCUSSION

The secretion of melatonin, a hormone of the pineal gland, is directly related to the circadian rhythm stimulated by darkness and suppressed by light. The postpeak melatonin level is less during the summer than during the winter.

In our earlier research on the psychological autopsy of completed suicide in children and adolescents, we found that suicide occurred more often during the dark part of the 24-hour cycle and also more often in the springtime, particularly the month of March (Shafii and Shafii 1982b). The suicide rate was higher in adolescents than in prepubescent children. Also, the suicide rate was four to five times higher in adolescent males. We found that 76% of the victims versus 24% of the control subjects had a major depressive disorder and/or dysthymic disorder as a primary or secondary diagnosis (Holden 1986; Shafii et al. 1984, 1985, 1988).

In searching for a biological marker for depression, Wetterberg (1983) and Beck-Friis et al. (1984) have found that adult depressed patients who were nonsuppressors on the DST had lower overnight serum melatonin levels than depressed patients who suppressed dexamethasone and a normal control group. This finding, along with our earlier observations, led to the study of the relationship between melatonin and depressive disorders in children and adolescents.

Ninety-six hospitalized patients ages 6–16 years participated in this study. Two or three bedtime and overnight urine samples were collected. Standardized instruments and structured interviews were used in diagnosis.

In radioimmunoassay of overnight urinary melatonin, we found that the mean melatonin level in children and adolescents with primary depression was significantly higher than in those who had secondary depression or those in the control group who had conduct and/or oppositional disorder. Simultaneous adjustment for age, sex, race, height, and weight did not have any effect on melatonin levels, nor did adjusting for the level of pubertal development or seasonal changes. On the other hand, some investigators found that nighttime serum melatonin level is lower in a heterogeneous group of depressed children and adolescents and also in some depressed adults. Could it be that in some depressive disorders the pineal gland functions bimodally in the form of hyperactivity or hypoactivity? Or perhaps that there are at least two types of depressive disorders in children and adolescents?—One form, primary depression, which may be associated with high melatonin, and the other, secondary depression, associated with melatonin levels similar to or lower than the control group. Whether melatonin levels are higher or lower in depressive disorders, there is a strong indication that the pineal gland plays an important role in the psychoneuroendocrinology of some types of depressive disorders in children and adolescents.

REFERENCES

Achenbach TM: The Child Behavior Profile, I: boys aged 6–11. J Consult Clin Psychol 46:478–488, 1978

Achenbach TM, Edelbrock CS: The Child Behavior Profile, II: boys aged 6–11 and 12–16. J Consult Clin Psychol 47:223–233, 1979

American Psychiatric Association: Diagnostic and Statistical Manual of Mental Disorders, 3rd Edition. Washington, DC, American Psychiatric Association, 1980

American Psychiatric Association: Diagnostic and Statistical Manual of Mental Disorders, 3rd Edition, Revised. Washington, DC, American Psychiatric Association, 1987

Anton-Tay F, Diaz JD, Fernandez-Guardiola A: On the effect of melatonin upon human brain: its possible therapeutic implications. Life Sci 10: 841–850, 1971

Arendt J, Paunier L, Sizonenko PC: Melatonin radioimmunoassay. J Clin Endocrinol Metab 40:347–350, 1975

Axelrod J, Weissbach H: Enzymatic O-methylation of N-acetylserotonin to melatonin. Science 131:1312, 1960

Beck AT: Hopelessness Scale. Philadelphia, PA, Center for Cognitive Therapy, 1978

Beck AT, Beamesderfer A: Assessment of depression: the depression inventory. Pharmacopsychiatra 7:151–169, 1974

Beck AT, Ward CH, Mendelson M, et al: An inventory for measuring depression. Arch Gen Psychiatry 4:561–571, 1961

Beck-Friis J, vonRosen D, Kjellman FJ, et al: Melatonin in relation to body measures, sex, age, season and the use of drugs in patients with major affective disorders and healthy subjects. Psychoneuroendocrinology 9:261–277, 1984

Carlson GA, Cantwell DP: Suicidal behavior and depression in children and adolescents. J Am Acad Child Adolesc Psychiatry 21:361–368, 1982

Carmen JS, Post RM, Buswell R, et al: Negative effects of melatonin on depression. Am J Psychiatry 133:1181–1186, 1976

Carroll BJ: The dexamethasone suppression test for melancholia. Br J Psychiatry 140:292–304, 1982a

Carroll BJ: Use of the dexamethasone suppression test in depression. J Clin Psychiatry 43:44–48, 1982b

Carroll BJ, Martin FIR, Davies BM: Resistance to suppression by dexamethasone of plasma 11-OCHS levels in severe depressive illness. Br Med J [Clin Res] 3:285–287, 1968

Carroll BJ, Curtis GC, Mendels J: Neuroendocrine regulation in depression, I: discrimination of depressed from nondepressed patients. Arch Gen Psychiatry 33:1051–1058, 1976

Carroll BJ, Feinberg M, Greden JF, et al: A specific laboratory test for the diagnosis of melancholia. Arch Gen Psychiatry 38:15–22, 1981

Cavallo A, Holt KG, Hejazi MS, et al: Melatonin circadian rhythm in childhood depression. J Am Acad Adolesc Child Psychiatry 26:395–399, 1987

Cramer H, Rudolph J, Consbruch U, et al: On the effects of melatonin on sleep and behavior in man, in Serotonin—New Vistas: Biochemistry and Behavioral and Clinical Studies (Advances in Biochemical Psychopharmacology, Vol 11). Edited by Costa E, Gessa GL, Sandler M. New York, Raven, 1974, pp 187–191

Crumley FE, Clevenger J, Steinfink D, et al: Preliminary report on the dexamethasone suppression test for psychiatrically disturbed adolescents. Am J Psychiatry 39:1062–1064, 1982

Cytryn L, McKnew DH, Logue M, et al: Biochemical correlates of affective disorders in children. Arch Gen Psychiatry 31:659–661, 1974

Extein I, Rosenberg G, Pottash ALC, et al: The dexamethasone suppression test in depressed adolescents. Am J Psychiatry 139:1617–1618, 1982

Feighner JP, Robins E, Guze SB, et al: Diagnostic criteria for use in psychiatric research. Arch Gen Psychiatry 26:57–62, 1972

Feinberg M, Carroll BJ: Biological "markers" for endogenous depression. Arch Gen Psychiatry 41:1080–1085, 1984

Geller B, Rogol AA, Knitter EF: Preliminary data on the dexamethasone suppression test in children with major depressive disorder. Am J Psychiatry 140:620–622, 1983

Ha H, Kaplan S, Foley C: The dexamethasone suppression test in adolescent psychiatric patients. Am J Psychiatry 141:421–423, 1984

Hamilton M: A rating scale for depression. J Neurol Neurosurg Psychiatry 23:56–62, 1960

Hamilton M: Clinical evaluation of depressions: clinical criteria and rating scales, including a Guttman Scale, in Depression: Behavioral, Biochemical, Diagnostic and Treatment Concepts. Edited by Gallant DM, Simpson GM. New York, Spectrum Publications, 1976, pp 155–179

Holden C: Youth suicide: new research focuses on a growing social problem. Science 233:839–841, 1986

Hsu LKG, Molcan K, Cashman MA, et al: The dexamethasone suppression test in adolescent depression. J Am Acad Child Adolesc Psychiatry 22:470–473, 1983

Hudson JI, Laffer PS, Pope HG: Bulimia related to affective disorder by family history and response to the dexamethasone suppression test. Am J Psychiatry 139:685–687, 1982

Hudson JI, Hudson MS, Rothschild AJ, et al: Abnormal results of dexamethasone suppression tests in nondepressed patients with diabetes mellitus. Arch Gen Psychiatry 41:1086–1089, 1984

Johnson LY, Reiter RJ: The pineal gland and its effects on mammalian reproduction. Progress in Reproductive Biology 4:116, 1978

Kashani JH, Husain A, Shekim WO, et al: Current perspectives on childhood depression: an overview. Am J Psychiatry 138:142–153, 1981

Kazdin AE, Rodgers A, Collins D: The Hopelessness Scale for Children: Psychosomatic Characteristics and Concurrent Validity. Pittsburgh, PA, University of Pittsburgh School of Medicine, Western Psychiatric Institute and Clinic, 1986

Khan AU: Biomedical profile of depressed adolescents. J Am Acad Child Adolesc Psychiatry 26:873–878, 1987

Kitay JJ: Pineal lesions and precocious puberty: a review. J Clin Endocrinol Metab 15:622–625, 1954

Klee SH, Garfinkle BD: Identification of depression in children and adolescents: the role of the dexamethasone suppression test. J Am Acad Child Adolesc Psychiatry 23:410–415, 1984

Kovacs M: Rating scales to assess depression in school-aged children. Acta Paedopsychiatry 46:305–315, 1981

Kovacs M, Beck AT: An empirical-clinical approach toward a definition of childhood depression, in Depression in Childhood: Diagnosis, Treatment, and Conceptual Models. Edited by Schuylterbrandt JC, Raskin A. New York, Raven, 1977, pp 1–25

Lenko H, Lang C, Aubert ML, et al: Hormonal changes in puberty, VII: lack of variation of daytime plasma melatonin. J Clin Endocrinol Metab 54:1056–1058, 1982

Lerner AB, Case JD, Takahashi Y, et al: Isolation of melatonin, the pineal gland factor that lightens melanocytes. Journal of the American Chemical Society 80:2587, 1958

Lerner AB, Case JD, Heinzelman RV: Structure of melatonin. Journal of the American Chemical Society 81:6084–6087, 1959

Lewy AJ, Wehr TA, Goodwin FK, et al: Light suppresses melatonin secretion in humans. Science 210:1267–1269, 1980

Lewy AJ, Kern HA, Rosenthal NE, et al: Bright artificial light treatment of a manic-depressive patient with a seasonal mood cycle. Am J Psychiatry 41:72–80, 1982

Lewy AJ, Sack RL, Miller LS, et al: Antidepressant and circadian phase shifting effects of light. Science 235:352–354, 1987

Livingston R, Reis CJ, Ringdahl IC: Abnormal dexamethasone suppression test results in depressed and nondepressed children. Am J Psychiatry 141:106–108, 1984

Lynch HJ, Wurtman RJ, Moskowitz MA, et al: Daily rhythm in human urinary melatonin. Science 187:169–171, 1975

McKnew DH, Cytryn L: Urinary metabolites in chronically depressed children. J Am Acad Child Adolesc Psychiatry 18:608–615, 1979

Meltzer HY, Fang VS: Cortisol determination and the dexamethasone suppression test. Arch Gen Psychiatry 40:501–505, 1983

Minitab Data Analysis Software, Minitab, Inc., Pond Laboratory, University Park, PA, 1985

Poznanski EO, Cook SC, Carroll BJ: A depression rating scale for children. Pediatrics 64:442–450, 1979

Poznanski EO, Carroll BJ, Banegas MC, et al: The dexamethasone suppression test in prepubertal depressed children. Am J Psychiatry 139:321–324, 1982

Poznanski EO, Grossman JA, Buchsbaum Y, et al: Preliminary studies of the reliability and validity of the Children's Depression Rating Scale. J Am Acad Child Adolesc Psychiatry 23:191–197, 1984

Puig-Antich J: Affective disorders in childhood: a review and perspective. Psychiatr Clin North Am 3:403–424, 1980

Puig-Antich J, Novacenko H, Goetz R, et al: Cortisol and prolactin responses to insulin-induced hypoglycemia in prepubertal major depressives during episode and after recovery. J Am Acad Child Adolesc Psychiatry 23:49–57, 1984a

Puig-Antich J, Novacenko H, Davies M, et al: Growth hormone secretion in prepubertal children, I: final report on response to insulin-induced hypoglycemia during a depressive episode. Arch Gen Psychiatry 41:455–460, 1984b

Puig-Antich J, Novacenko H, Davies M, et al: Growth hormone secretion in prepubertal children with major depression, III: response to insulin-induced hypoglycemia after recovery from a depressive episode and in a drug-free state. Arch Gen Psychiatry 41:471–475, 1984c

Reiter RJ: The pineal gland and gonadal development in male rats and hamsters. Fertil Steril 19:1009–1017, 1968

Robbins DR, Alessi NE, Yanchyshyn GW, et al: Preliminary report on the dexamethasone suppression test in adolescents. Am J Psychiatry 139:942–943, 1982

Robbins DR, Alessi NE, Yanchyshyn GW, et al: The dexamethasone suppression test in psychiatrically hospitalized adolescents. J Am Acad Child Adolesc Psychiatry 22:467–469, 1983

Robins L, Helzer JE, Ratcliff KS, et al: Validity of the Diagnostic Interview Schedule, Version II: DSM-III diagnoses. Psychol Med 12:855–857, 1982

Rosenthal NE, Sack DA, Gillin C, et al: Seasonal affective disorder: a description of the syndrome and preliminary findings with light therapy. Arch Gen Psychiatry 41:72–80, 1984

Rosenthal NE, Sack DA, Gillin C, et al: Antidepressant effects of light in seasonal affective disorder. Am J Psychiatry 142:163–170, 1985

Scheffé H: The Analysis of Variance. New York, John Wiley, 1959, pp 68–72

Shafii M, Shafii SL: Depression in infancy, childhood, and adolescents: failure in human contact, sadness, and withdrawal, in Pathways of Human Development: Normal Growth and Emotional Disorders in Infancy, Childhood, and Adolescence. New York, Thieme-Stratton, 1982a, pp 77–95

Shafii M, Shafii SL: Self-destructive, suicidal behavior, and completed suicide, in Pathways of Human Development: Normal Growth and Emotional Disorders in Infancy, Childhood, and Adolescence. New York, Thieme-Stratton, 1982b, pp 164–180

Shafii M, McCue A, Ice JF, et al: The development of an acute short-term inpatient child psychiatric setting: a pediatric-psychiatric model. Am J Psychiatry 136:427–429, 1979

Shafii M, Whittinghill JR, Dolen DC, et al: Psychological reconstruction of completed suicide in childhood and adolescence, in Suicide in the Young. Edited by Sudak HS, Ford AB, Rushford NB. Boston, MA, John Wright, PSG, 1984, pp 271–294

Shafii M, Carrigan S, Whittinghill JR, et al: Psychological autopsy of completed suicide in children and adolescents: a comparative study. Am J Psychiatry 142:1061–1064, 1985

Shafii M, Steltz-Lenarsky J, Derrick AM, et al: Comorbidity of mental disorders in the post-mortem diagnosis of completed suicide in children and adolescents. J Affective Disord 15:227–233, 1988

Shivers BD, Yochim JM: Pineal serotonin N-acetyltransferase activity in the rat during the estrous cycle and in response to light. Biology Reprod 21:385–391, 1979

Silman LE, Leone RM, Hooper RJL, et al: Melatonin, the pineal gland and human puberty. Nature 282:301–303, 1979

Spitzer RL, Endicott J, Robins E: Research Diagnostic Criteria: rationale and reliability. Arch Gen Psychiatry 35:773–782, 1978

Swartz CM, Dunner FJ: Dexamethasone suppression testing of alcoholics. Arch Gen Psychiatry 39:1309–1312, 1982

Tamarkin L, Westrom WK, Hamill AI, et al: Effects of melatonin on the reproductive systems of male and female Syrian hamsters. Endocrinology 99:1534–1541, 1976

Tamarkin L, Baird CJ, Almeida OFX: Melatonin: a coordinating signal for mammalian reproduction? Science 227:714–720, 1985

Tanner JM: Growth at Adolescence, 2nd Edition. Oxford, Blackwell Scientific Publishers, 1962

Weller EB, Weller RA, Fristad MA, et al: The dexamethasone suppression test in hospitalized prepubertal depressed children. Am J Psychiatry 141:290–291, 1984

Wetterberg L: Melatonin in humans: physiological and clinical studies. J Neural Transm [Suppl] 13:289–310, 1978

Wetterberg L: The relationship between the pineal gland and the pituitary-adrenal axis in health, endocrine and psychiatric conditions. Psychoneuroendocrinology 8:75–80, 1983

Wetterberg L, Eriksson O, Friberg Y, et al: A simplified radioimmunoassay for melatonin and its application to biological fluids: preliminary observations on the half-life of plasma melatonin in man. Clin Chim Acta 86:169–177, 1978

Wetterberg L, Beck-Friis J, Kjellman BF, et al: Circadian rhythms in melatonin and cortisol secretion in depression, in Frontiers in Biochemical and Pharmacological Research in Depression. Edited by Usdin E, Åsberg M, Bertilsson L, et al. New York, Raven, 1984, pp 197–205

Wurtman RJ, Axelrod J, Fischer JE: Melatonin synthesis in the pineal gland: effect of light mediated by the sympathetic nervous system. Science 143:1328–1330, 1964

Zetin M, Potkin S, Urbancheck M: Melatonin in depression. Psychiatric Annals 17:676–681, 1987

Chapter 5

Melatonin and Circadian Rhythms in Bipolar Mood Disorder

Aimee Mayeda, M.D.
John Nurnberger, Jr., M.D., Ph.D.

Chapter 5

Melatonin and Circadian Rhythms in Bipolar Mood Disorder

Bipolar mood disorder is marked by recurrent cycles of mania, depression, and normal mood. The cyclic nature of mood changes has prompted some investigators to suggest that mood disorders may be caused by disturbed circadian rhythms (Wehr et al. 1983). Several other clinical features of mood disorders lend support to this idea. Patients in both the manic and depressive states typically manifest profound disturbances in body functions that normally have circadian rhythms, including sleep, motor activity, appetite, and endocrine function.

Melatonin is secreted in a precise circadian rhythm. It appears to play a role in regulating other physiologic rhythms in mammals (see Chapters 1 and 2). Investigations of disturbances in melatonin secretion in bipolar illness may shed light on the nature of this illness and its relationship to circadian rhythm disturbances.

CIRCADIAN RHYTHMS AND THEIR RELATION TO LIGHT

Circadian rhythms are physiological and behavioral variations that recur every 24 hours, coordinating internal events with the environment. For example, body temperature in most diurnal mammals is maximal during the early evening and lowest in the morning before waking; cortisol secretion peaks in the morning shortly before waking, with minimal secretion at night (Wever 1979). The secretion of many other hormones, including melatonin, prolactin, and growth hormone, follow circadian cycles. More than independent variations, circadian rhythms are coordinated and interdependent, permitting organisms to prepare in advance for environmental events (Aschoff 1965). Obvious circadian behaviors like waking and sleeping are contingent on other circadian rhythms such as the inhibition of diuresis and urination during sleep (Healy 1987).

Circadian rhythms are endogenous and self-sustaining, able to persist in the absence of external input (Aschoff 1965). Cultured chick pineal cells in constant darkness release melatonin in a rhythmic pattern that has a period very close to 24 hours (Robertson and Takahashi 1988a, 1988b). When humans are deprived of environmental time cues (zeitgebers) such as dawn, dusk, or social schedules, oscillations in body temperature and sleep continue with a period close to 25 hours (Wever 1979). Central nervous system (CNS) lesioning experiments indicate that the suprachiasmatic nucleus (SCN) of the hypothalamus is the circadian pacemaker (Moore and Klein 1974; Rusack and Zucker 1979). Isolated rat SCN in vitro retains circadian rhythms of single-unit firing rates (Gillette and Prosser 1988).

Because the intrinsic rhythm in normal humans is closer to 25 hours than to 24 hours, it must be entrained, or readjusted, daily to synchronize with the external day-night cycle. The major zeitgeber for entraining circadian rhythms in most plant and animal species is the environmental light-dark cycle (Aschoff 1965). Light entrains the endogenous circadian rhythm to the 24-hour cycle via the retina and the retinohypothalamic pathway to the SCN in mammals, including humans (Moore and Klein 1974; Sadun et al. 1984). The cholinergic agonist carbachol produces an effect on the SCN similar to the effect of light, suggesting that some of the connections between the retinohypothalamic tract and the SCN are cholinergic (Zatz and Brownstein 1979). The effect of light is blocked by α-bungarotoxin (Zatz and Brownstein 1981), which suggests that a subtype of nicotinic receptor is involved.

In most animals, circadian rhythms can be manipulated by changing the light-dark cycle. Bright light is also a zeitgeber in humans when the intensity is about 2,500 lux or greater, higher than normal artificial lighting (Lewy et al. 1980) (see Chapter 6). Social cues are also important zeitgebers for humans (Wever 1985). This may explain why we can adjust to working at night or eating at unusual hours (Healy 1987).

MELATONIN RELEASE IN ANIMALS AND HUMANS

The secretion of melatonin by the pineal gland exhibits circadian rhythmicity in almost all mammals, including humans. Melatonin secretion is normally very low during the day (Arendt 1985) and maximal during the night (see Chapter 2). In humans, daytime levels are barely detectable (< 5 pg/ml), and nocturnal peaks range between

20 and 140 pg/ml (Lewy and Markey 1978). Although there are marked interindividual differences in melatonin levels, there is high individual consistency (Arendt 1985).

Light is the primary environmental influence on melatonin secretion, and its influence is to suppress melatonin production. A multisynaptic pathway conveys information about the photoperiod from the SCN to the pineal gland. The pathway appears to include the paraventricular nucleus of the hypothalamus, the intermediolateral cell column of the spinal cord, and the superior cervical ganglion (Bittman and Lehman 1987; Moore 1978; Patrickson and Smith 1987). From there, sympathetic output innervates the pineal via β-adrenergic receptors on the pinealocyte (see Chapter 1). Melatonin synthesis is inhibited by β-blockers and stimulated by β-adrenergic receptor activation in all mammalian species except sheep (Arendt 1985).

Changes in the light-dark cycle can change the pattern of melatonin secretion in duration, phase, or amplitude (Lewy 1984). In animals, melatonin appears to transmit circadian rhythm information from the SCN to entrain physiologic rhythms (Redman et al. 1983). Administered melatonin is soporific in humans and some animals (Lerner and Nordlund 1978; Marczynski et al. 1964). A function of evening melatonin secretion may be to cause sedation, thereby entraining rest to darkness. Injected melatonin entrains rest-activity cycles in free-running rats (Redman et al. 1983) and speeds entrainment to a new cycle (Murakami et al. 1983). On the other hand, pigs with normal circadian activity cycles have little circadian variation in their melatonin levels (Reiter et al. 1987).

The best evidence that melatonin transmits photoperiod information comes from research on seasonal or annual rhythms, particularly rhythms of sexual function. Seasonal rhythms in behavior and physiology are exhibited by many animals, including humans. The photoperiod, or interval between dawn and dusk, varies with the time of year and triggers physiologic and behavior changes related to seasonal breeding, growth, hibernation, and migration (Arendt 1985). Hamsters and sheep with pineal lesions are unable to coordinate their breeding activities with the seasons (Arendt 1985; Bittman et al. 1983).

Administered melatonin induces the same effects as photoperiod changes on seasonal cycles in some experimental animals. Sheep develop estrus in late autumn when the photoperiod is short. The duration of high plasma levels of melatonin in sheep corresponds to the length of darkness (Arendt 1985). Infusion of melatonin during anestrus into pinealectomized ewes to produce the long plasma melatonin profiles typical of winter nights led to hormone changes usually seen in estrus (Bittman et al. 1983). Melatonin was given orally to male white-tailed deer in April to produce melatonin blood levels typical of June. The deer developed hair molt, antler calcification, rutting behavior, and elevations of plasma prolactin, follicle-stimulating hormone, and testosterone 60 days before the onset of these changes in untreated deer populations (Bubenik et al. 1986).

There is little evidence as yet that melatonin has an important physiologic role in humans. A few apparently normal humans have low to undetectable levels of melatonin (Arendt 1985). Patients chronically treated with β-blockers show suppressed melatonin secretion without ill effects (Cowen et al. 1983, 1985).

At one time, it was thought that melatonin modulated puberty in humans. Melatonin levels decline as luteinizing hormone rises in puberty, which suggests that melatonin is antigonadotropic and inhibits sexual maturation (Waldhauser and Dietzel 1985). Furthermore, pineal tumors are associated with abnormal pubertal development (Klein 1984). However, recent data from Waldhauser et al. (1988) are most consistent with the interpretation that the fall in plasma melatonin in young men at puberty is a function of increasing body size, rather than sexual maturation (see Chapter 4). Melatonin levels decrease with chronological age (Iguchi et al. 1982; Sack et al. 1986).

Bright light can shift the phase of melatonin secretion in humans (Broadway et al. 1987). The photoperiodic control of melatonin makes it a potential marker of circadian rhythms. Lewy (1983) has suggested use of the dim-light melatonin onset as a marker of circadian rhythm phase and period (see Chapter 6).

BIPOLAR DISORDER AND CIRCADIAN RHYTHM DISTURBANCE

Both the manic and depressive states of bipolar disorder are marked by profound changes in many bodily functions that are under circadian control, such as sleep, awakening, appetite, motor activity, and endocrine activity. Depressive symptoms also frequently demonstrate a circadian rhythm, most severe in the early morning and almost absent in the evening. Many studies demonstrate disruptions of circadian rhythms in manic-depressive patients (Wehr et al. 1983). These findings suggest several hypotheses about the role circadian rhythm disturbances play in bipolar illness, including internal desynchronization, phase advance, and genetic vulnerability.

Internal Desynchronization in Bipolar Illness

Bunney et al. (1972) and Sitaram et al. (1978) noted that bipolar patients showed a marked reduction in sleep on the night before they switched from depression into mania. Wehr and Goodwin (1980) noted that at the beginning of a manic episode, 9 of 10 manic-depressive patients had one or more 48-hour rest-activity cycle. Patients remained awake with no subjective sense of drowsiness for one to four alternate nights. The investigators were intrigued by the similarities between the rest-activity cycles of these patients and those of normal subjects deprived of zeitgebers.

Under normal conditions, the various circadian rhythms in the body are synchronized with each other and with the external dark-light cycle (Aschoff 1965). When normal humans are deprived of zeitgebers, their rest-activity cycles and temperature cycles remain synchronized with a period near 25 hours for the first few weeks. For some subjects, however, the period of the rest-activity cycle lengthens to around 45 hours, whereas the period of the temperature cycle, which also appears to be coordinated with the cycles of rapid eye movement (REM) sleep and cortisol excretion, remains 25 hours. The result is "internal desynchronization." The two rhythms go in and out of phase, generating repeating 25-hour cycles occasionally interrupted by a 48-hour cycle. During the switch from short to long cycles, the subject may remain awake for 30 hours or more with no subjective drowsiness (Wever 1979).

Investigators have noted internal desynchronization in persons traveling across time zones and in shift workers (Arendt and Marks 1982). Jet lag or shift work can cause sleep disturbances with features of endogenous depression such as weight loss, anorexia, irritability, and lack of energy (Akerstedt and Gillberg 1981; Arendt and Marks 1982). It is not clear why some workers adjust to changing shifts without difficulty whereas others never adjust.

The similarity between the 48-hour cycles of bipolar patients at the beginning of a manic episode and those in normal subjects with internal desynchronization suggested that bipolar patients were internally desynchronized. Kripke et al. (1978) and others hypothesized that depression or mania results from beat phenomena generated when the two rhythms are in and out of phase.

Sleep-deprivation studies provided some support for the theory that internal desynchronization causes changes in mood states. Forty of 45 patients with major depression showed remission of depressive symptoms after sleep deprivation, with complete remission in 16 patients after a single night of sleep deprivation. Results were similar in a group of 12 bipolar patients (Pflug 1976). Wehr et al. (1982) asked nine rapid-cycling bipolar patients to simulate the 48-hour cycle of internal desynchronization by remaining awake for 40 hours. Eight of the nine patients switched out of depression, and seven developed mania or hypomania. In a number of patients, recovery sleep failed to reverse the hypomanic state. Kripke et al. (1978) found further evidence consistent with this theory. They saw temperature rhythms in several bipolar patients in a normal environment advance earlier each day. This suggested that the period of their temperature rhythm was less than 24 hours. In some of these patients, lithium lengthened the period of the temperature rhythm, suggesting that lithium may prevent manic or depressed episodes by preventing internal desynchronization.

Some bipolar patients appear to have internal desynchronization, and, at the time of a mood switch, their sleep-wake cycle mimics that of normal subjects with internal desynchronization. However, evidence is lacking that temperature and sleep-wake cycles are desynchronized at the time of a mood switch. Wehr et al. (1985) saw no evidence for desynchronization of the two rhythms in a bipolar patient cycling rapidly between depression and mania. It is also not clear why internal desynchronization causes severe mood changes of mania and depression in bipolar patients but not in normal subjects.

Phase Shift in Bipolar Disorder

Early morning awakening is a prominent feature of depression in some unipolar and bipolar patients. This has suggested to several investigators that the phase of the temperature-REM cycle was shifted earlier relative to the rest-activity cycle in these individuals. Wehr and Goodwin (1981) reviewed the evidence for phase advance in depression and found advances in several measures, including REM sleep, temperature, cortisol, and neurotransmitter metabolites (see Chapters 6 and 8).

Several studies have found similar phase advances in bipolar patients (Sack et al. 1987). Wehr et al. (1980) noted that patients who were either manic or depressed had a 3- to 6-hour advance in the peak of 3-methoxy-4-hydroxyphenyl glycol (MHPG) secretion. Hartmann (1968) found a phase change in REM latency, the period from the time sleep begins until the time REM begins. In five of six bipolar patients, REM latency was state dependent: slightly increased in patients in the manic state and slightly decreased in patients in the depressed state. Four of seven bipolar patients spontaneously advanced their times of awakening as a depressive episode ended (Wehr et al. 1979).

Wehr et al. (1979) hypothesized that if the phase advance of the temperature-REM cycle relative to the rest-activity cycle was causing mood disorders, then changing sleep patterns to realign the phase of these cycles would restore normal mood. Several groups advanced the sleep period 5–6 hours in bipolar patients by altering their normal sleep period of 11 P.M.–7 A.M. to 5 P.M.–1 A.M. Many patients had remission of their depressive episodes, and the remissions lasted 1 week or more (see review in Sack et al. 1985, 1987). Partial sleep deprivation in the second half of the night was as effective an antidepressant as total sleep deprivation (Schilgen and Tolle 1980), whereas partial sleep deprivation in the first half of the night appeared to have little effect (see review in Sack et al. 1985). Partial sleep deprivation in the second half of the night is similar to phase advance of the sleep cycle in that both procedures cause a 5- to 6-hour advance in the time of awakening.

These studies suggest that bipolar patients have a phase advance of some cycles during the depressed state and perhaps a phase delay in manic states. Lewy et al. (1985) hypothesized that bipolar patients have increased sensitivity to light in the morning and that this caused the observed phase advance of circadian rhythms. However, most of the studies of phase advance have focused on unipolar patients. Phase advance of circadian cycles in bipolar patients in both the depressed and manic states needs further study.

Genetic Factors

Bipolar patients may have a genetic predisposition for disrupted circadian rhythms or increased susceptibility to mood disorder should circadian rhythm disruption occur. As noted above, internal desynchronization rarely precipitates severe affective changes such as mania or depression in normal subjects. Ehlers et al. (1988) suggested that life events disrupt daily routines, causing circadian rhythm disruption, but whether this disruption leads to major depression depends on vulnerability factors such as genetic susceptibility.

There is evidence for a genetic diathesis, or predisposition, for bipolar disorder. On average, 25% of first-degree relatives of bipolar patients will have unipolar or bipolar illness at some point in their lives (Gershon et al. 1982). Two single major gene forms of bipolar mood disorder were described, one linked to DNA markers on the short arm of chromosome 11 (Egeland et al. 1987) and one linked to markers on the X chromosome (Baron et al. 1987). However, reanalysis of the pedigree in Egeland's study has excluded linkage to the loci on chromosome 11 (Kelsoe et al. 1989). Many bipolar families do not have the X chromosome marker.

The nature of the genetic diathesis for bipolar disorder is unclear, but it may well be an abnormality in circadian rhythm regulation. Animal studies have demonstrated that genetic factors determine circadian rhythms. Konopka and Benzer (1971) produced three "clock mutants" in Drosophila with abnormal circadian rhythms. One had a 19-hour period, one had a 28-hour period, and one was arrhythmic. Mice of the inbred strain C57BL/6J have no detectable melatonin secretion (Ebihara et al. 1986) and abnormalities in the amplitude and phase of their temperature rhythm (Connolly and Lynch 1983). Ralph and Menaker (1988) found evidence that a mutation at a single autosomal locus caused a period of 20 hours in mutant golden hamsters.

Genetic factors also influence melatonin secretion. Wetterberg et al. (1983) studied urinary melatonin in a group of 107 humans from 23 nuclear families. Complex segregation analysis showed that melatonin production may be regulated by an additive major gene (see Chapter 3).

Susceptibility to rhythm disruption also appears to have a genetic component. Ralph and Menaker (1988) noted that although wild-type hamsters cannot entrain if their endogenous and entraining cycle periods differ by more than an hour, many clock mutants could entrain to cycles different by 2 hours or more from their internal clock.

The nature of the genetic diathesis for bipolar disorder is unclear; it may involve an increased susceptibility to disruption of circadian rhythms. Animal data suggest that a predisposition to disrupted rhythms can be inherited. Alternatively, bipolar patients may have a genetic susceptibility to mood changes when circadian rhythms are disrupted. Certain shift workers seem to be more vulnerable than others to mood changes associated with circadian rhythm disruption. Bipolar patients may be especially vulnerable. Wehr et al. (1982) noted that rapid-cycling bipolar patients are more sensitive to the antidepressant effects of sleep deprivation than unipolar depressed patients. Kripke et al. (1978) suggested that bipolar patients have a genetic predisposition that causes desynchronization to be exacerbated once it occurs.

MELATONIN SECRETION IN BIPOLAR ILLNESS

Most of the studies that have examined melatonin levels in patients with mood disorders have focused on patients with unipolar depression (see Chapters 3 and 4). Interindividual variation in melatonin secretion and single-time-point melatonin measurements complicated analysis of these studies. A low level at a single time point can result from either a phase shift or a change in amplitude. Thompson et al. (1988) noted that many published studies had not tested for possible covariates that might affect melatonin secretion, such as age, sex, menstrual status, season of testing, height, and weight.

Psychoactive drugs also cause changes in melatonin secretion. Lithium treatment in rats causes a decrease in amplitude and a phase shift in melatonin secretion (Seggie and Werstiuk 1985; Yocca et al. 1983). Antidepressant drugs have both increased and decreased melatonin secretion in humans (Miles and Philbrick 1988).

Investigations of melatonin secretion in bipolar disorder included measurement of melatonin levels, phase shift of the melatonin secretion curve, and light suppression of melatonin secretion.

Melatonin Amplitude in Patients With Mood Disorder

In contrast to numerous studies of melatonin in unipolar depressed patients, only two studies focus on the amplitude of melatonin levels in bipolar patients. Beck-Friis et al. (1985b) studied 12 euthymic bipolar patients along with 12 euthymic unipolar patients, 30 acutely ill unipolar depressive patients, and 33 control subjects. The euthymic bipolar patients had significantly lower maximum melatonin levels than the control subjects. Euthymic unipolar depressive patients and acutely ill unipolar patients with abnormal dexamethasone suppression tests also showed low maximal melatonin levels. The authors hypothesized that low melatonin levels were a trait marker for the subgroup of depressed patients with abnormalities of the hypothalamic-pituitary-adrenal axis (see Chapter 3).

Lewy et al. (1979) found increased melatonin secretion during both day and night in four manic bipolar patients: 24-hour melatonin secretion was twice that of unmatched control subjects. Three of four had diminished melatonin secretion when they were depressed. From this, Lewy hypothesized in 1985 that the amplitude of melatonin secretion is state dependent and reflects CNS β-adrenergic function.

Lewy's hypothesis is consistent with the studies of melatonin secretion amplitude in unipolar depressive patients where the trend for decreased melatonin in depressed patients is striking. In 9 of 11 patient groups studied, depressed patients have lower than normal amplitude of melatonin secretion (Beck-Friis et al. 1985a; Boyce 1985; Branchey et al. 1982; Brown et al. 1985; Claustrat et al. 1984; Mendlewicz et al. 1979; Nair et al. 1984; Wetterberg 1983; Wirz-Justice and Arendt 1979). Two studies showed no difference (Jimmerson et al. 1977; Thompson et al. 1988) (see Chapter 3, Table 3-1).

Taken together, these data suggest that the amplitude of melatonin secretion is state dependent in bipolar patients, as Lewy hypothesized.

However, much more data, especially on patients in the manic state, are needed to confirm this hypothesis.

Phase Shift in the Melatonin Cycle

The evidence for phase-shifted melatonin secretion in mood disorders is also inconclusive but suggestive. Lewy et al. (1979) found that the phase of maximum melatonin secretion was advanced in four manic patients relative to control subjects. They also noted that one subject had her peak melatonin secretion during the day, 180° out of phase with control subjects. During this time, her activity-rest cycle was completely disorganized and she napped sporadically both day and night. When her melatonin secretion pattern was in phase with the light-dark cycle, her activity-rest cycle was relatively normal. Beck-Friis et al. (1985b) did not evaluate phase shift in melatonin secretion in the 12 euthymic bipolar patients they examined.

In studies of unipolar depressive patients, Nair et al. (1984) noted not only decreased peak melatonin levels in six depressed patients, but also delayed onset of the nocturnal melatonin rise and phase advance of the melatonin peak. However, Claustrat et al. (1984) and Brown et al. (1985) reported no melatonin phase shift in the groups they examined.

Light Suppression Studies

When humans are exposed to light during the night, melatonin secretion decreases within 30–60 minutes. The brighter the light, the greater the observed decline in plasma melatonin levels (Lewy et al. 1980). The intensity of ordinary room light is usually 200-300 lux and rarely over 500 lux, whereas the intensity of sunlight on a sunny afternoon is 100,000 lux (Lewy 1983). Several studies suggest that manic-depressive patients and their relatives have increased sensitivity to the melatonin-suppressing effects of light.

Lewy et al. reported in 1981 that four bipolar patients had 50% suppression of plasma melatonin levels when exposed to 500 lux of light at 2 A.M. and almost complete suppression of melatonin when exposed to 1,500 lux. In six healthy, sex-matched control subjects, there was no suppression of melatonin when they were exposed to 500 lux and only 40% suppression in two control subjects who were exposed to 1,500 lux. Two of the bipolar patients were manic and two were depressed at the time of the study (Lewy et al. 1985).

In follow-up studies, 15 euthymic bipolar patients and 26 control subjects were evaluated (Lewy et al. 1985; Nurnberger et al. 1988), and supersensitivity to light in well-state bipolar patients was demonstrated. Five hundred lux of light decreased melatonin levels

62% on average for the 11 patients and 28% for the 24 control subjects in the first study (Lewy et al. 1985). Taken together with the earlier data from acutely ill bipolar patients, this suggested that augmented melatonin suppression was a trait marker for bipolar disorder.

A study of high-risk offspring of bipolar patients (Nurnberger et al. 1988) showed parallels between suppression of melatonin by 500 lux of light and risk of mood disorder. Patients with two ill parents had on average 73% suppression of melatonin, whereas patients with one ill parent had 57% suppression, and control subjects had 45% suppression. The risk of mood disorder paralleled the percentage of melatonin suppression in five groups of subjects: psychiatrically screened control subjects, unscreened control subjects, patients with one parent ill, patients with two parents ill, and bipolar patients (Table 5-1; Figure 5-1). Follow-up studies are in progress to determine whether melatonin suppression has value in predicting genetic vulnerability to mood disorder in these families.

The nature of the hypothesized vulnerability leading to hypersensitivity to light requires further clarification. The inhibitory effects of light on the SCN may be mediated by nicotinic cholinergic mechanisms; hypersensitivity of these receptors in bipolar patients is possible. The projections from the superior cervical ganglion to the pineal gland that stimulate melatonin production are β-adrenergic; bipolar patients may have subsensitivity of postsynaptic receptors or increased sensitivity of presynaptic, inhibitory receptors. Alternatively, other neurons in the pathway from the retina to the pineal may be involved. A study is now in progress to replicate the findings of

Table 5-1.   Relationship between morbid risk of mood disorder and melatonin suppression

Group	Estimated morbid risk (%)	High melatonin suppression (%) ($\geq$ 0.84 SD above mean)
Screened controls	5–9	15
Unscreened controls	10–15	21
One parent ill	18–15	33
Two parents ill	35–55	57
Patients	100	91

Note. The morbid risk estimates are based on the mean age of the group and the family study data of Gershon et al. (1982, 1987). Percentage of high melatonin suppression is calculated from the group data in Figure 5-1. The cutoff point is the point of maximum separation between unscreened control subjects and patients (see Lewy et al. 1985; Nurnberger et al. 1988).

supersensitivity to light in euthymic bipolar patients and to clarify the response to β-adrenergic blockers.

Buchsbaum et al. (1973) demonstrated greater rates of increased amplitude of average evoked responses to increasing intensities of light (augmentation) in bipolar patients, whether in the depressed or manic phase. Although another mechanism may mediate both phenomena, these data indicate bipolar patients have increased sensitivity to light which mediates increased melatonin suppression.

SUMMARY

Patients with bipolar mood disorder have abnormalities of their circadian rhythms—the physiological and behavioral variations that recur daily and coordinate internal physiologic events with the environment. At the beginning of a manic episode, certain patients have one or more 48-hour sleep-wake cycles (Wehr and Goodwin 1980), and some have temperature cycles that advance earlier every day (Kripke et al. 1978).

Experimentally manipulating the circadian rhythms of bipolar patients can cause mood changes. A number of rapid-cycling bipolar patients deprived of sleep for one night switched out of depression

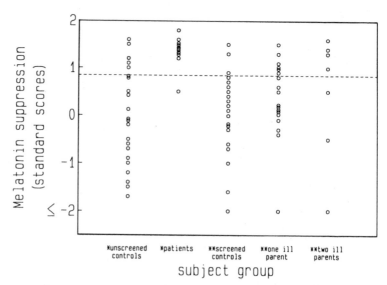

Figure 5-1.   Melatonin suppression in bipolar patients, control subjects, and high-risk offspring. *Data from Lewy et al. 1985. **Data from Nurnberger et al. 1988.

and developed mania (Wehr et al. 1982). Advancing the sleep period has been an effective antidepressant in bipolar patients (Sack et al. 1987).

Melatonin secretion and bipolar mood disorder seem to be subject to genetic control. A genetic predisposition for bipolar mood disorder may involve increased susceptibility to circadian rhythm disruption or susceptibility to changes in mood after rhythm disruption. This may involve increased sensitivity to light (Lewy et al. 1985).

Melatonin secretion is under circadian control but is abnormal in some bipolar patients. The phase of melatonin secretion may be abnormal (Lewy et al. 1979), and it is suggested that peak melatonin secretion is state dependent, decreased in depressed and euthymic states, and increased in mania (Beck-Friis et al. 1985b; Lewy et al. 1979). Several studies suggest that bipolar patients and their relatives have increased sensitivity to the melatonin-suppressing effects of light (Lewy et al. 1985; Nurnberger et al. 1988) and that the risk of mood disorder may be related to this sensitivity to light. Melatonin secretion may be a useful tool for investigating the genetic vulnerability to bipolar disorder.

REFERENCES

Akerstedt T, Gillberg M: Sleep disturbances and shift work. Advances in the Biosciences 3:127–137, 1981

Arendt J: The pineal hormone melatonin in seasonal and circadian rhythms, in Circadian Rhythms in the Central Nervous System. Edited by Redfern PH, Campbell IC, Davies JA, et al. London, Macmillan, 1985, pp 15–24

Arendt J, Marks V: Physiologic changes underlying jet lag. Br Med J [Clin Res] 284:144–146, 1982

Aschoff J: Circadian rhythms in man. Science 148:1427–1432, 1965

Baron M, Risch N, Hamburger R, et al: Genetic linkage between X-chromosome markers and bipolar affective illness. Nature 326:289–295, 1987

Beck-Friis J, Kjellman BF, Aperia B, et al: Serum melatonin in relation to clinical variables in patients with major depressive disorder and a hypothesis of a low melatonin syndrome. Acta Psychiatr Scand 71:319–330, 1985a

Beck-Friis J, Kjellman BF, Ljungren J-G, et al: The pineal gland and melatonin in affective disorders, in The Pineal Gland: Endocrine Aspects (Advances in the Biosciences, Vol 53). Edited by Brown GM, Wainwright SD. Oxford, Pergamon, 1985b

Bittman EL, Lehman MN: Paraventricular neurons control hamster photoperiodism by a predominantly uncrossed descending pathway. Brain Res Bull 19:687–694, 1987

Bittman EL, Dempsey RJ, Karsch FJ: Pineal melatonin secretion drives the reproductive response to daylength in the ewe. Endocrinology 113:2276–2283, 1983

Boyce PM: 6-Sulphatoxymelatonin in melancholia. Am J Psychiatry 142:125–127, 1985

Branchey L, Weinberg U, Branchey M, et al: Simultaneous study of 24-hour patterns of melatonin and cortisol secretion in depressed patients. Neuropsychobiology 8:225–232, 1982

Broadway J, Arendt J, Folkard S: Bright light phase shifts the human melatonin rhythm during the Antarctic winter. Neuroscience Letters 79:185–189, 1987

Brown R, Kocsis JH, Caroff S, et al: Differences in nocturnal melatonin secretion between melancholic depressed patients and control subjects. Am J Psychiatry 142:811–816, 1985

Bubenik GA, Smith PS, Schams D: The effect of orally administered melatonin on the seasonality of deer pelage exchange, antler development, LH, FSH, prolactin, testosterone, T_3, T_4, cortisol, and alkaline phosphatase. J Pineal Res 3:331–349, 1986

Buchsbaum M, Landau S, Murphy D, et al: Average evoked response in bipolar and unipolar affective disorders: relationship to sex, age of onset, and monoamine oxidase. Biol Psychiatry 7:199–212, 1973

Bunney WE, Murphy DL, Goodwin FK, et al: The "switch process" in manic-depressive illness. Arch Gen Psychiatry 27:295–302, 1972

Claustrat B, Chazot G, Brun J, et al: A chronological study of melatonin and cortisol secretion in depressed subjects: plasma melatonin, a biochemical marker in major depression. Biol Psychiatry 19:1215–1228, 1984

Connolly MS, Lynch CB: Classical genetic analysis of circadian body temperature rhythms in mice. Behav Genet 13:491–500, 1983

Cowen PJ, Frazer S, Sammons R, et al: Atenolol reduces plasma melatonin concentration in man. Br J Clin Pharmacol 15:579–581, 1983

Cowen PJ, Bevan JS, Gosden B, et al: Treatment with β-adrenoceptor blockers reduces plasma melatonin concentration. Br J Clin Pharmacol 19:258–260, 1985

Ebihara S, Marks T, Hudson DJ, et al: Genetic control of melatonin synthesis in the pineal gland of the mouse. Science 231:491–493, 1986

Egeland JA, Gerhard DS, Pauls DL, et al: Bipolar affective disorders linked to DNA markers on chromosome 11. Nature 325:783–787, 1987

Ehlers CL, Frank E, Kupfer DJ: Social zeitgebers and biological rhythms. Arch Gen Psychiatry 45:948–952, 1988

Gershon ES, Hamovit JH, Guroff JJ, et al: A family study of schizoaffective, bipolar I, bipolar II, unipolar, and normal control probands. Arch Gen Psychiatry 39:1157–1167, 1982

Gershon ES, Hamovit JH, Guroff JJ, et al: Birth-cohort changes in manic and depressive disorders in relatives of bipolar and schizoaffective patients. Arch Gen Psychiatry 44:314–319, 1987

Gillette MU, Prosser RA: Circadian pacemaker properties are retained by isolated suprachiasmatic nuclei in vitro. Society for Neuroscience Abstracts 14:385, 1988

Hartmann E: Longitudinal studies of sleep and dream patterns in manic-depressive patients. Arch Gen Psychiatry 19:312–329, 1968

Healy D: Rhythm and blues: neurochemical, neuropharmacological and neuropsychological implications of a hypothesis of circadian rhythm dysfunction in the affective disorders. Psychopharmacology 93:271–285, 1987

Iguchi H, Kato K, Ibayashi H: Age-dependent reductions in serum melatonin concentrations in healthy human subjects. J Clin Endocrinol Metab 55:27–29, 1982

Jimerson DC, Lynch HJ, Post RM, et al: Urinary melatonin rhythms during sleep deprivation in depressed patients and normals. Life Sci 20:1501–1508, 1977

Kelsoe JR, Ginns EI, Egeland JA, et al: Re-evaluation of the linkage relationship between chromosome 11p loci and the gene for bipolar affective disorder in Old Order Amish. Nature 342:238–243, 1989

Klein DC: Melatonin and puberty. Science 224:6, 1984

Konopka RJ, Benzer S: Clock mutants of *Drosophila melanogaster*. Proc Natl Acad Sci USA 68:2112–2116, 1971

Kripke DF, Mullaney DJ, Atkinson M, et al: Circadian rhythm disorders in manic-depressives. Biol Psychiatry 13:335–350, 1978

Lerner AB, Nordlund JJ: Melatonin: clinical pharmacology. J Neural Transm [Suppl] 13:339–347, 1978

Lewy AJ: Biochemistry and regulation of mammalian melatonin production, in The Pineal Gland. Edited by Relkin R. New York, Elsevier, 1983, pp 77–128

Lewy AJ: Human melatonin secretion (II): a marker for the circadian system and the effects of light, in Neurobiology of Mood Disorder. Edited by Post RN, Ballenger JC. Baltimore, MD, Williams & Wilkins, 1984, pp 215–226

Lewy AJ, Markey SP: Analysis of melatonin in human plasma by gas chromatography negative chemical ionization mass spectrometry. Science 201:741–743, 1978

Lewy AJ, Wehr TA, Gold PW, et al: Plasma melatonin in manic-depressive illness, in Catecholamines: Basic and Clinical Frontiers, Vol 2. Edited by Usdin E, Kopin IJ, Barchas J. New York, Pergamon, 1979

Lewy AJ, Wehr TA, Goodwin FK, et al: Light suppresses melatonin secretion in humans. Science 210:1267–1269, 1980

Lewy AJ, Wehr TA, Goodwin FK, et al: Manic-depressive patients may be supersensitive to light. Lancet 1:383–384, 1981

Lewy AJ, Nurnberger JI, Wehr TA, et al: Supersensitivity to light: possible trait marker for manic-depressive illness. Am J Psychiatry 142:725–727, 1985

Marczynski TJ, Yamaguchi N, Ling GM, et al: Sleep induced by the administration of melatonin (5-methoxy-N-acetyltryptamine) to the hypothalamus in unrestrained cats. Experientia 20:435–437, 1964

Mendlewicz J, Linkowski P, Branchey L, et al: Abnormal 24 hour pattern of melatonin secretion in depression. Lancet 2:1362, 1979

Miles A, Philbrick DRS: Melatonin and psychiatry. Biol Psychiatry 23:405–425, 1988

Moore RY: Neural control of pineal function in mammals and birds. J Neural Transm [Suppl] 13:47–58, 1978

Moore RY, Klein DC: Visual pathways and the central neural control of a circadian rhythm in pineal serotonin N-acetyltransferase activity. Brain Res 71:17–33, 1974

Murakami N, Hayafuji C, Sasaki Y, et al: Melatonin accelerates the reentrainment of the circadian adrenocortical rhythm in inverted illumination cycle. Neuroendocrinology 36:385–391, 1983

Nair NPV, Hariharasubramanian N, Pilapil C: Circadian rhythm of plasma melatonin in endogenous depression. Prog Neuropsychopharmacol Biol Psychiatry 8:715–718, 1984

Nurnberger JI, Berrettini W, Tamarkin L, et al: Supersensitivity to melatonin suppression by light in young people at high risk for affective disorder. Neuropsychopharmacology 1:217–223, 1988

Patrickson JW, Smith TE: Possible suprachiasmatic nucleus→spinal cord pathways. Society for Neuroscience Abstracts 13:1106, 1987

Pflug B: The effect of sleep deprivation on depressed patients. Acta Psychiatr Scand 53:148–158, 1976

Ralph MR, Menaker M: A mutation of the circadian system in golden hamsters. Science 241:1225–1227, 1988

Redman J, Armstrong S, Ng KT: Free-running activity rhythms in the rat: entrainment by melatonin. Science 219:1089–1091, 1983

Reiter RJ, Britt JH, Armstrong JD: Absence of a nocturnal rise in either norepinephrine, N-acetyltransferase, hydroxyindole-O-methyltransferase or melatonin in the pineal gland of the domestic pig kept under natural environmental photoperiods. Neuroscience Letters 81:171–176, 1987

Robertson LM, Takahashi JS: Circadian clock in cell culture, I: oscillation of melatonin release from dissociated chick pineal cells in flow-through microcarrier culture. J Neurosci 8:12–21, 1988a

Robertson LM, Takahashi JS: Circadian clock in cell culture, II: in vitro photic entrainment of melatonin oscillation from dissociated chick pineal cells. J Neurosci 8:22–30, 1988b

Rusack B, Zucker I: Neural regulation of circadian rhythms. Physiol Rev 59:449–526, 1979

Sack DA, Nurnberger JI, Rosenthal NE, et al: Potentiation of antidepressant medications by phase advance of the sleep-wake cycle. Am J Psychiatry 142:606–608, 1985

Sack DA, Rosenthal NE, Parry BL, et al: Biological rhythms in psychiatry, in Psychopharmacology, The Third Generation of Progress. Edited by Meltzer HY. New York, Raven, 1987, pp 669–685

Sack RL, Lewy AJ, Erb DL, et al: Human melatonin production decreases with age. J Pineal Res 3:379–388, 1986

Sadun AA, Schaechter JD, Smith LE: A retinohypothalamic pathway in man: light mediation of circadian rhythms. Brain Res 302:371–377, 1984

Schilgen B, Tolle R: Partial sleep deprivation as therapy for depression. Arch Gen Psychiatry 37:267–271, 1980

Seggie J, Werstiuk ES: Lithium and melatonin rhythms: implications for depression, in The Pineal Gland: Endocrine Aspects (Advances in the Biosciences, Vol 53). Edited by Brown GM, Wainwright SD. Oxford, Pergamon, 1985, pp 333–338

Sitaram N, Gillin JC, Bunney WE: The switch process in manic-depressive illness. Acta Psychiatr Scand 58:267–278, 1978

Thompson C, Franey C, Arendt J, et al: A comparison of melatonin secretion in depressed patients and normal subjects. Br J Psychiatry 152:260–265, 1988

Waldhauser F, Dietzel M: Daily and annual rhythms in human melatonin secretion: role in puberty control. Ann NY Acad Sci 453:205–214, 1985

Waldhauser F, Weiszenbacher G, Tatzer E, et al: Alterations in nocturnal serum melatonin levels in humans with growth and aging. J Clin Endocrinol Metab 66:648–652, 1988

Wehr TA, Goodwin FK: Desynchronization of circadian rhythms as a possible source of manic-depressive cycles. Psychopharmacol Bull 16:19–20, 1980

Wehr TA, Goodwin FK: Biological rhythms in psychiatry, in American Handbook of Psychiatry. Edited by Arieti S, Brodie HKH. New York, Basic Books, 1981, pp 46–67

Wehr TA, Wirz-Justice A, Goodwin FK, et al: Phase advance of the circadian sleep-wake cycle as an antidepressant. Science 206:710–713, 1979

Wehr TA, Muscettola G, Goodwin FK: Urinary 3-methoxy-4-hydroxyphenylglycol circadian rhythm. Arch Gen Psychiatry 37:257–263, 1980

Wehr TA, Goodwin FK, Wirz-Justice A, et al: 48-hour sleep-wake cycles in manic-depressive illness. Arch Gen Psychiatry 39:559–565, 1982

Wehr TA, Sack D, Rosenthal N, et al: Circadian rhythm disturbances in manic-depressive illness. Federal Proceedings 42:2809–2813, 1983

Wehr TA, Sack DA, Duncan WC, et al: Sleep and circadian rhythms in affective patients isolated from time cues. Psychiatry Res 15:327–339, 1985

Wetterberg L: The relationship between the pineal gland and the pituitary-adrenal axis in health, endocrine and psychiatric conditions. Psychoneuroendocrinology 8:75–80, 1983

Wetterberg L, Iselius L, Lindsten J: Genetic regulation of melatonin excretion in urine. Clin Genet 24:399–402, 1983

Wever RA: The Circadian System of Man: Results of Experiments Under Temporal Isolation. New York, Springer-Verlag, 1979

Wever RA: Use of light to treat jet lag: differential effects of normal and bright artificial light on human circadian rhythms. New York Academy of Science 453:282–304, 1985

Wirz-Justice A, Arendt J: Diurnal, menstrual cycle and seasonal indole rhythms in man and their modification in affective disorders, in Biological Psychiatry Today. Edited by Obiols J, Ballus C, Gonzalez Monclus E, et al. Amsterdam, Elsevier, 1979

Yocca FD, Lynch V, Friedman E: Effect of chronic lithium treatment on rat pineal rhythms: N-acetyltransferase, N-acetylserotonin and melatonin. J Pharmacol Exp Ther 226:733–737, 1983

Zatz M, Brownstein MJ: Intraventricular carbachol mimics the effect of light on the circadian rhythm in the rat pineal gland. Science 203:358–361, 1979

Zatz M, Brownstein MJ: Injection of alpha-bungarotoxin near the suprachiasmatic nucleus blocks the effects of light on nocturnal pineal enzyme activity. Brain Res 213:438–442, 1981

PART III

Light Therapy and the Pineal Gland

Chapter 6

Bright Light, Melatonin, and Winter Depression: The Phase-Shift Hypothesis

Alfred J. Lewy, M.D., Ph.D.
Robert L. Sack, M.D.
Clifford M. Singer, M.D.

Chapter 6

Bright Light, Melatonin, and Winter Depression: The Phase-Shift Hypothesis

Over the centuries, many connections of mood to light and the seasons have been made. Even songwriters and poets have made astute observations on this topic. Given such a long-standing familiarity with seasonal changes in light and mood, it is surprising that bright-light treatment of winter depression was not discovered until recently.

Only a few decades ago, animal research began to elucidate the role of light (specifically day length) in the regulation of seasonal rhythms (Zucker 1988). Over the past three decades, the effects of light on circadian rhythms and the pineal gland were gradually described (Fiske et al. 1960; Klein and Weller 1972; Quay 1964; Wurtman et al. 1963). About 10 years ago, scientists would have been completely prepared to link seasonal rhythms in humans to annual changes in environmental light, except that studies in the late 1970s suggested that humans were uniquely unresponsive to the light-dark cycle.

Indeed, before 1980, the prevailing point of view was that humans lacked many of the responses to light that are ubiquitous among other species (Klein 1979). One source of this thinking was from chronobiologists who believed that, despite the knowledge that light entrains the circadian rhythms of almost all other species (Aschoff 1981a), it was less important than social cues in entraining human circadian rhythms (Wever 1979). This thinking was also reinforced by the uniformly negative findings that resulted from attempts to suppress human nighttime melatonin production with light (Arendt

We thank C. Simonton for help in preparing this manuscript and G. Clarke, M. Cardoza, M. Blood, V. Bauer, F. Colby, S. Beck, J. Authier, D. Wesche, K. Sparlin, and J. Peterson for help with these studies. These studies were supported by NIMH Grants MH-40161 (A.J.L.) and MH-00703 (A.J.L.).

1978; Jimerson et al. 1977; Lynch et al. 1977; Vaughan et al. 1979; Weitzman et al. 1978; Wetterberg 1978). The problem with these studies was that apparently humans require much brighter light than do most other species to convincingly demonstrate these responses.

Wehr and Rosenthal (1989) have tracked down almost all relevant published material regarding light treatment of winter depression, and Kern and Lewy (1990) have made additions and corrections to this review. In this chapter, we examine major steps taken in recognizing winter depression and the use of bright-light therapy for treatment.

BRIGHT LIGHT AND SUPPRESSION OF MELATONIN IN HUMANS

The effect of bright light in suppression of melatonin in humans was discovered in a self-experiment. Shortly after returning to Washington, D.C., after a 2-week stay in Australia, the investigator (A.J.L.) measured his morning plasma melatonin levels with a newly developed negative chemical ionization gas chromatography–mass spectrometry assay (Lewy and Markey 1978). His melatonin levels were low, when they should have been high—given that the Australian nighttime increase should still have been occurring during the Washington, D.C., day. This finding suggested that sunlight was suppressing his melatonin production.

Next, the sleep-wake cycles and light-dark cycles of two normal control subjects were shifted to a schedule on which they slept in the dark between 3 and 11 A.M. for 1 week (Lewy et al. 1980). This was done to shift their "nighttime" melatonin production so that the suppressant effect of sunlight could be tested. At the end of the week, their plasma melatonin levels were measured, and a 4-hour delay was documented: levels were still high at 11 A.M. On day 8, the subjects were awakened at 7 A.M. and exposed to sunlight. Melatonin levels promptly decreased. We concluded that sunlight was capable of suppressing melatonin production in humans.

Intensity was then chosen as the most important difference between sunlight and ordinary room light (Lewy et al. 1980). When six control subjects were awakened between 2 and 4 A.M., bright (2,500 lux) light caused the same suppression as dimmer light had been documented to cause in other species (Figure 6-1, *left*). Dimmer light (500 lux) did not cause much suppression of melatonin production in these subjects. Light of 1,500-lux intensity suppressed melatonin production to an intermediate extent (Figure 6-1, *right*). We speculated that, perhaps because of routine exposure to bright (outdoor) light,

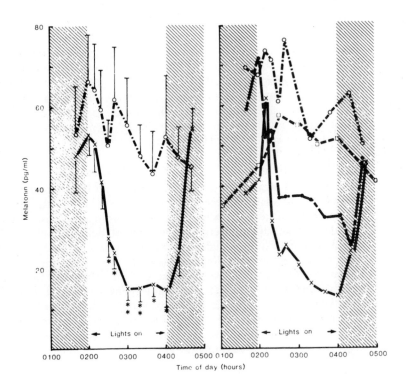

Figure 6-1. *Left,* effect of light on melatonin secretion. Each point represents mean (± SE) concentration of melatonin for six subjects. Paired *t* test comparing exposure to 500 lux with exposure to 2,500 lux was performed for each data point. Two-way analysis of variance with repeated measures and Newman-Keuls statistic for comparison of means showed significant differences between 2:30 and 4 A.M. (**P < .5;**P < .01*). *Right,* effect of different light intensities on melatonin secretion. Average values for two subjects are shown. ○, 500 lux; X, 2,500 lux; ●, 1,500 lux; □, asleep in dark. Reprinted from Lewy et al. 1980, with permission from publisher. Copyright 1980 by the American Association for the Advancement of Science.

humans have become relatively insensitive to indoor light compared with laboratory animals who were born and raised indoors. Evidence for this speculation has since been documented (Reiter et al. 1983).

As mentioned above, chronophysiologists had concluded that light was not an important zeitgeber (environmental time cue) compared with social cues (Wever 1979), despite the ubiquity of these responses in other species (Aschoff 1981a). Our finding that human melatonin production could be suppressed with bright light prompted us to speculate that humans might have many of the same circadian and seasonal responses to light observed in other species, except that bright light would be required to convincingly demonstrate these in humans (Lewy et al. 1980). This is the first pivotal paper on this topic.

BRIGHT LIGHT AND WINTER DEPRESSION

The above findings suggested that humans could be responding to natural (bright) daylight, relatively unperturbed by ordinary room light. That is, extending winter days with ordinary-intensity light would not make day length constant year-round. Before our discovery of suppression of human nighttime melatonin production by bright light, scientists could not logically conceive of seasonal rhythms in humans regulated by day length, because the differences between indoor (dim) and outdoor (bright) light intensity were not thought to be of physiologic importance. It was thought that either humans do not have biological rhythms that responded to light or that they do have this potential but live in a light-dark cycle that does not differ year-round, thus not providing the cues for these rhythms to change during the year.

Seasonal rhythms have not been documented to a great extent in humans (Aschoff 1981b). However, almost all of the circadian rhythms known in animals are present in humans (Aschoff 1981a). Nevertheless, our first application of the finding of bright-light suppression of melatonin was to treat a patient who had a seasonal pattern in recurrent mood swings (Lewy et al. 1982): generally, as the days shortened in the winter, he became depressed, and, as the days lengthened in the spring, he came out of these depressions (Lewy et al. 1982; Rosenthal et al. 1983). Because animals measure day length by the time interval between the dawn and dusk light-dark transitions (Aschoff 1981b), we exposed our first patient to 3 hours of bright light twice a day between 6 and 9 A.M. for 10 days to produce a "spring" day length. After 4 days of this light exposure schedule, the patient began to switch out of his depression (Lewy et al. 1982).

This case report is what many would regard as the second pivotal paper of the modern phase of research on light therapy of winter depression. If there are historical forces at work here, one is clearly the long-standing interest of Herbert E. Kern in trying to understand and to treat, albeit unsuccessfully, his own depression (Kern and Lewy 1990). The other historical force is rooted in more than 30 years of animal studies on seasonal rhythms, melatonin production, and the effects of light. This case report opened up the specific area of light therapy for winter depression and perhaps for other biological rhythm disorders, whereas the first pivotal paper (Lewy et al. 1980) opened up the general area of light and human biological rhythms and led directly to the second pivotal paper (Lewy et al. 1982).

With the successful treatment of Mr. Kern, the current field of light therapy of winter depression began. It should also be mentioned that Mr. Kern had previously contacted Peter S. Mueller, M.D., in 1976, after which several antidepressant and mood-stabilizing drug regimens were tried unsuccessfully (H.E. Kern, personal communication). Mueller had become interested in seasonal depression and the influence of temporarily moving to a more southerly climate. In August of 1980, he treated a patient with artificial full-spectrum light of unspecified intensity (Mueller and Allen 1984).

The third pivotal paper was the first study of a group of patients with winter depression by Rosenthal et al. (1984). The experimental design in this study was based on the first two studies: bright light was used as the "active" treatment compared with presumedly biologically less active dim-light exposure (Lewy et al. 1980), again scheduled in the early morning and late afternoon to increase day length (Lewy et al. 1982). Rosenthal et al. (1984) discovered that many more patients had seasonal affective disorder (winter depression) than was previously thought and described the general clinical characteristics of these patients. However, there is some disagreement over whether the majority of these patients are bipolar (as suggested in the Rosenthal et al. article) or unipolar (which many would say is the prevailing point of view today).

Types of Placebo Controls

The study by Rosenthal et al. (1984) was also the first attempt to use a double-blind placebo control; based on our earlier finding (Lewy et al. 1980), dim light was used as a placebo treatment. Patients responded to the bright light but not to the dim light. Unfortunately, it is not clear if the dim light served as a plausible placebo control because patients were generally aware of which was the bright light and which was the dim light. Furthermore, a sampling of treatment expectations indicated that most patients thought that the bright light would be more antidepressant than the dim light. Consequently, even in this early study, dim light could not be regarded as a true placebo control. Subsequent studies comparing bright light with dim light have the same methodological problem. Most patients probably think that the bright light would be more effective than the dim light (James et al. 1985; Rosenthal et al. 1985).

Therefore, the first successful attempt at comparing a biologically effective light treatment to a plausible placebo treatment may have been the first morning versus evening light crossover study (Lewy et al. 1987a). As assessed by a posttreatment expectation questionnaire, patients did not expect the morning light to be more antidepressant than the evening light. Light treatments were of equal intensity and duration. Patients were told that some would respond to morning light, some to evening light, some to both, and some to neither. Patients generally missed the absence of evening light rather than morning light in the winter. When asked which time they would prefer for light therapy, they generally picked evening light, because it did not involve awakening earlier, which they were reluctant to do. For these reasons, as well as because of data from questionnaires assessing pre- and posttreatment expectations, we think that evening bright light continues to be a plausible placebo treatment control for morning light.

THE PHASE-SHIFT HYPOTHESIS

At about the same time we were conducting our first light-treatment study, Kripke (1981) began to treat patients with major melancholic depression with bright light, exposing patients to bright light in the morning. This schedule of exposure was based on the theory that there was a critical interval in the morning that required bright-light exposure (Kripke 1984). We, on the other hand, thought that these patients should be exposed to bright light in the evening (Lewy et al. 1983), if—as hypothesized by Kripke et al. (1978), Papousek (1975), and Wehr et al. (1979)—these patients had abnormally phase-advanced circadian rhythms. According to our hypothesis, evening bright light would provide a corrective phase delay (Lewy et al. 1983).

Our thinking was based on phase-response curves (PRCs) in animals (Decoursey 1964; Pittendrigh and Daan 1976). The PRC is the relationship between the direction and magnitude of a phase shift and the time of day when the light exposure occurs. Light exposure during the subjective day has relatively little phase-shifting effect. Light exposure during the first half of subjective night causes phase delays (shifts to a later time); light exposure during the subjective day causes phase advances (shifts to an earlier time). The closer to the middle of the night, the greater the magnitude of these phase shifts.

Also, in the middle of the night, there is an inflection point that separates the greatest phase delays from the greatest phase advances.

We had some preliminary evidence that humans had similarly shaped PRCs (Lewy et al. 1983), except that they required bright light for these responses. Wever et al. (1983) demonstrated circadian rhythm effects of bright light in humans. Lewy et al. (1984, 1985a) phase-shifted circadian rhythms by shifting the (bright) light-dark cycle while holding the activity-rest cycle constant (see below). Based on our hypothesized PRC for humans, we began treating with evening light patients who had phase-advanced circadian rhythms, the same type that Kripke (1981) is treating with morning bright light. Our results were mixed. The early morning awakening responded well: after 4 days of evening bright light, patients slept throughout the night. However, the antidepressant response was more variable. Kripke et al. (1989) have since switched over to the evening bright-light exposure. They, too, report variable effects but have concluded that there is a statistically significant antidepressant response.

At present, the use of bright light in the treatment of major melancholic (nonseasonal) depression is still not nearly as effective as the use of bright light in the treatment of winter depression. After our first case report, many more patients have since been similarly and successfully treated. Most investigators agree that the light has to be sufficiently intense and of a sufficient duration; however, there is still some controversy over whether the timing of the light exposure is critical (Terman et al. 1989).

Morning Versus Evening Bright-Light Exposure

The Bethesda group has consistently maintained that the timing of the light exposure is not critical (James et al. 1985; Rosenthal et al. 1985; Wehr et al. 1986). On the other hand, our group has for several years maintained that bright light is—for most patients—more effective in the treatment of winter depression when scheduled in the morning rather than in the evening (Lewy et al. 1984). Both groups have long been aware that, as opposed to patients with major melancholic depression, winter depressive patients have morning hypersomnia (i.e., they complain of difficulty getting up in the morning). Based on this observation, the Bethesda group began to treat these patients with evening light (James et al. 1985; Rosenthal et al. 1985), because they thought that patients would comply better with light therapy scheduled in the evening since they would not have to awaken earlier, which they were reluctant to do. Based on the same observation of morning hypersomnia, we began to treat these patients with morning light and to compare this treatment with evening light.

We hypothesized that the morning hypersomnia in these patients indicated abnormally phase-delayed circadian rhythms that would respond best to a corrective phase advance which would occur after morning light exposure (Lewy et al. 1983, 1984).

Thus, the morning light treatment initially proposed by Kripke (1981) for phase-advanced major melancholic depression and the evening light treatment at one time proposed by the Bethesda group (James et al. 1985; Rosenthal et al. 1985) for winter depression were opposite to the treatments we proposed for these disorders (Lewy et al. 1983, 1984). Our approach to the treatment of these disorders was based on a unified theory called "phase typing" (Lewy et al. 1984, 1985b). What we mean by phase typing is that before treating an individual with bright light, one should decide whether light exposure should be scheduled in the morning or in the evening. Patients thought to have abnormally phase-delayed circadian rhythms should be treated first with bright light scheduled in the morning, in order to provide a corrective phase advance. Patients thought to have abnormally phase-advanced circadian rhythms should be treated first with bright light in the evening, in order to provide a corrective phase delay.

When we describe a rhythm as phase advanced or phase delayed, we mean not only with respect to real time but also with respect to sleep. In other words, we are describing the phase of endogenous circadian rhythms (such as melatonin, cortisol, and temperature) relative to sleep. There is an irony here. For example, in phase-delayed mood disorders, endogenous circadian rhythms are phase delayed relative to sleep. In these disorders, sleep may be slightly phase delayed relative to real time along with the other endogenous circadian rhythms. However, sleep is actually phase advanced relative to the other endogenous circadian rhythms.

Nevertheless, sleep phase is often used clinically for phase typing, based on the observation that relative to real time all circadian rhythms—including sleep—are shifted in the same direction, even though sleep may be shifted to a greater or lesser extent than the other circadian rhythms. One example is that of delayed sleep-phase syndrome, in which the typical patient cannot fall asleep before 3 A.M. and often sleeps until 11 A.M. In the case of advanced sleep-phase syndrome, the typical patient sleeps between 9 P.M. and 3 A.M.

MELATONIN: A CIRCADIAN PHASE MARKER

Phase typing becomes more difficult if an individual falls asleep early and awakens late, or falls asleep late and awakens early. In these cases, we usually use sleep-offset time rather than sleep-onset time to mark circadian phase, because it is less influenced by psychological factors such as anxiety and boredom. In any event, the best circadian phase marker is melatonin, because sleep and the endogenous circadian rhythms of cortisol and temperature are influenced by extraneous factors such as stress and activity. Melatonin is not affected by stress and activity, only by bright light (Lewy 1983).

As mentioned above, we showed that shifting the (bright) light-dark cycle could shift human circadian rhythms, holding the sleep-wake cycle constant (Lewy et al. 1984, 1985a). In a study of four normal volunteers who slept for 15 days between 11 P.M. and 6 A.M., "dusk" was advanced for 1 week from between 7:30 P.M. and 9 P.M. to 4 P.M. On the first night of advanced dusk, the onset of melatonin production advanced 1.5 hours earlier, whereas the offset of melatonin did not change (Figure 6-2). Over the next 2 days, the onset remained at a stable phase position (Figure 6-3); however, by the end of the week, it had advanced one more hour, as did the offset (Figure 6-2). For the 2nd week, "dawn" was delayed from between 6 A.M. and 7:30 A.M. to 9 A.M. There was no change in the onset or the offset until the end of the week, when both had delayed 1 hour (Figure 6-4).

These data provide evidence for the hypothesis of a PRC in humans (Lewy et al. 1983). Bright light in the evening appears to be causing a phase delay of the melatonin rhythm, whereas bright light in the morning appears to be causing a phase advance. Some investigators think that there are separate oscillators for the melatonin onset and offset in rodents (Illnerová and Vanecek 1982). Our data, and their data (the duration of melatonin production in humans does not change during the year [Illnerová et al. 1985]), suggest that *functionally* humans have only one oscillator.

These data also provide evidence for a suppressant effect of bright light. After advancing dusk, there was an immediate advance in the onset, which remained at a stable phase position for 1 or 2 more days, whereas there was no immediate advance in the offset. We have interpreted these results to mean that removing bright light in the evening unmasks the correct phase of the melatonin onset. Therefore, the melatonin onset is an ideal phase marker, providing that blood is drawn under dim-light conditions after 5 or 6 P.M.

The dim-light melatonin onset (DLMO) is a clearly demarcated marker for circadian phase. We currently recommend that light intensity be below 50 lux (below the intensity of light comfortable for reading). Occasionally, we use goggles to reduce ordinary room light below this intensity (Figure 6-5). We have been particularly insistent on reducing light intensity as much as possible for the

DLMO ever since we found that some control subjects will suppress their melatonin production to a significant degree in response to 500 lux of light exposure between 2 and 4 A.M. (Lewy et al. 1985d).

We have used these findings to study putative chronobiologic sleep and mood disorders. As mentioned above, we expect patients who have a chronobiologic sleep or mood disorder to be of either the phase-advance type or the phase-delay type. Patients of the phase-advance type should preferentially respond to evening light; patients of the phase-delay type should preferentially respond to morning light. We have proposed that patients with chronobiologic sleep disorders should have all of their circadian rhythms—including

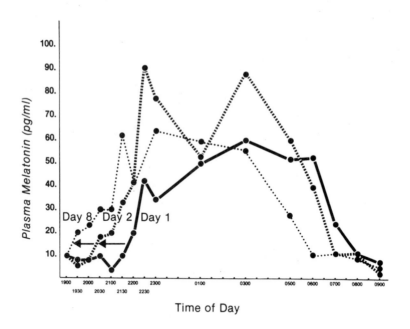

Time of Day

Figure 6-2. Mean nighttime plasma melatonin levels for four subjects on day 1 (*solid line*) of study (when dusk was between 7:30 and 9 P.M. and dawn was between 6 and 7:30 A.M.) and on days 2 (*dashed line*) and 8 (*dotted line*), the 1st and 7th days, respectively, after dusk was advanced to 4 P.M. (while dawn was held constant). Sleep was held constant between 11 P.M. and 6 A.M. throughout study (see Figures 6-4 and 6-5). Reprinted from Lewy et al. 1985a, with permission from the publisher.

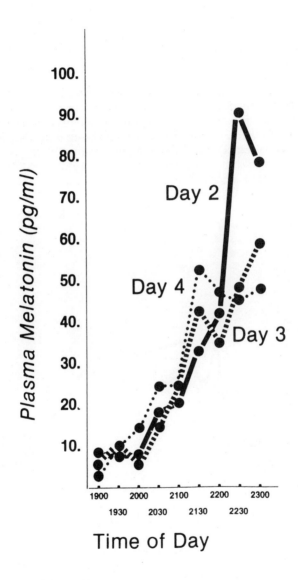

Figure 6-3.   Mean plasma melatonin levels between 7 and 11 P.M. on days 2 (*solid line*), 3 (*dashed line*), and 4 (*dotted line*). Reprinted from Lewy et al. 1985a, with permission from publisher.

sleep—phase shifted to the same extent, or perhaps sleep is more phase shifted than the other circadian rhythms (Lewy et al. 1988). Similar to what Wehr et al. (1979) have proposed (for nonseasonal depression), we think that in all chronobiologic mood disorders, sleep is not as phase shifted as the other circadian rhythms, creating what we call a phase-angle disturbance.

Treatment of chronobiologic sleep disturbances is straightforward. Patients with delayed sleep-phase syndrome respond to morning light: after a few days of bright light scheduled as soon as they awaken or slightly before their previous day's wake-up time, they are able to gradually advance all of their circadian rhythms including sleep, which is allowed to shift to the desired phase (Lewy et al. 1983). Similarly, patients with advanced sleep-phase syndrome respond to evening light (Lewy et al. 1985c).

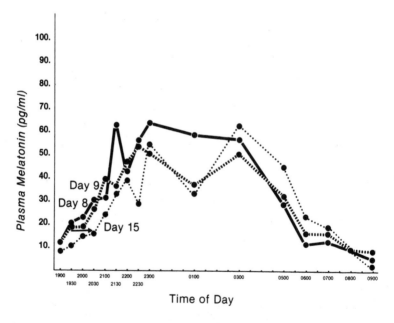

Figure 6-4. Mean nighttime plasma melatonin levels on day 8 (*solid line*), the 7th day of advanced dusk, and on days 9 (*dashed line*) and 15 (*dotted line*), the 1st and 7th days, respectively, after dawn was delayed to 9 A.M. (while dusk was held constant). Reprinted from Lewy et al. 1985a, with permission from publisher.

TREATMENT OF WINTER DEPRESSION

Treatment of chronobiologic mood disturbances is not so straightforward. For this reason, we have devoted most of our investigations to the study of patients with winter depression. As mentioned above, we thought that the fact that these patients have difficulty arising in the morning when depressed in the winter indicated a phase-delay type of circadian rhythm disturbance. This is not intuitively obvious. For example, although many of these patients sleep later in the winter, many of them also go to bed earlier. Nevertheless, we decided to

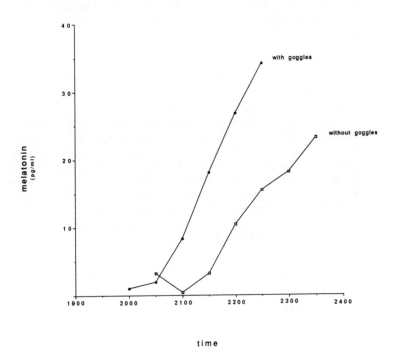

Figure 6-5. Melatonin onsets in sighted subject under two different lighting conditions during blood drawing. Without goggles = 100–300 lux (ordinary room light). With goggles = less than 50 lux (difficult to read fine print). In this individual, ordinary room light was sufficiently intense to cause apparent phase delay in melatonin onset. We are currently recommending that dim-light melatonin onsets be performed under dimmest possible light.

investigate the possibility that winter depression was a chronobiologic mood disturbance and specifically hypothesized that for most patients, winter depression is a phase-delay type of circadian rhythm disturbance (Lewy et al. 1984). We further hypothesized that they became more delayed in the winter because of the later dawn and that they would preferentially respond to bright light scheduled in the morning because it would provide a corrective phase advance.

We tested this hypothesis in the winter of 1984–1985 (Lewy et al. 1987a). Eight patients and seven control subjects were studied over a 4-week protocol. The 1st week was a baseline adaptation week. Patients and control subjects were in dim light between 5 P.M. and 8 A.M. They slept between 10 P.M. and 6 A.M. for all 4 weeks of the study. At week 2, half were randomly assigned to morning (6–8 A.M.) bright (2,500 lux) light, and half were assigned to evening (8–10 P.M.) bright light. At week 3, they were crossed over to the other light schedule. Thus, when scheduled for morning bright light, bright light was avoided in the evening and vice versa. At the 4th week, they were exposed to bright light at both times.

Depression ratings significantly declined at the end of the week of morning bright light compared with those at the end of the baseline week and the end of the week of evening bright light (Figure 6-6). There were no other statistically significant differences. However, depression ratings at the end of the week of morning plus evening light were intermediate between those after morning light alone and those after evening light alone, as if the combination of light exposures counteract each other when evening light is scheduled sufficiently late. As mentioned above, patients did not expect morning light to be more antidepressant than evening light. Consequently, the evening light served as a plausible placebo control treatment for these patients.

On the 1st day of the study, patients' DLMOs were significantly delayed compared with those of the control subjects (Figure 6-7). More importantly, their DLMOs were also significantly delayed compared with those of the control subjects at the end of the baseline week, thus reflecting an intrinsic abnormality in the circadian system of the patients. That is, the patients' DLMOs were not delayed because their sleep offset and therefore morning light exposure might have been delayed.

Morning light advanced the DLMOs, and evening light delayed them. This was true for patients and control subjects, except that patients advanced more in response to morning light and delayed less in response to evening light than did control subjects. These findings

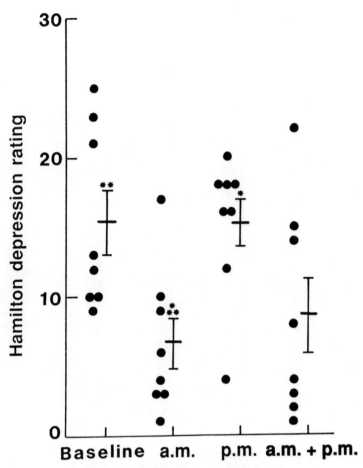

Figure 6-6. Individual and average 21-item Hamilton depression ratings (±SE) for eight patients with winter depression for each of 4 weeks of study. Analysis of variance for repeated measures indicated significant (*P* = .026) difference between treatments. Only paired *t* tests comparing week of morning (A.M.) light and baseline week (**P* = .004) and comparing week of A.M. light and week of evening (P.M.) light (*P* = .045) were significant. Average depression ratings for seven control subjects were 3.0 ± 0.9 at baseline, 2.4 ± 0.3 for A.M. light, 6.1 ± 1.6 for P.M. light, and 4.3 ± 0.9 for A.M. + P.M. light. Reprinted from Lewy et al. 1987a, with permission from publisher. Copyright 1987 by the American Association for the Advancement of Science.

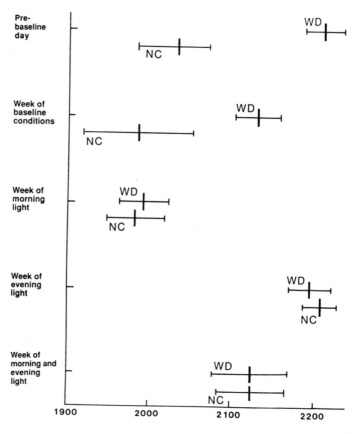

Figure 6-7. Average melatonin onset times ($\pm$ SE) for normal control subjects (NC) and patients with winter depression (WD). $n = 6$–8, except $n = 4$ for prebaseline melatonin values. Analysis of variance for repeated measures indicated significant difference between treatments for WD ($P = .001$) and NC ($P = .009$). Significant paired t tests for WD were baseline versus A.M. ($P = .001$), baseline versus P.M. ($P = .012$), and A.M. versus P.M. ($P = .001$). Significant paired t tests for NC were baseline versus A.M. + P.M. ($P = .039$), A.M. versus P.M. ($P = .004$), and A.M. versus A.M. + P.M. ($P = .003$). Melatonin onset times of WD were delayed compared with those of NC at prebaseline ($P = .02$) and at baseline ($P = .05$) (Student's t test). Reprinted from Lewy et al. 1987a, with permission from publisher. Copyright 1987 by the American Association for the Advancement of Science.

suggest that the PRCs of the patients were delayed compared with the control subjects.

Because the patients' DLMOs returned to baseline after the week of evening light treatment, the evening-light depression ratings serve as a measure of the nonspecific (placebo) component of the antidepressant response to 2 hours of bright-light exposure. Even if the evening light had delayed the DLMOs to a time later than baseline, evening light would still provide a valid control for testing the phase-shift hypothesis, because any worsening due to a phase delay is nonetheless a test of the same hypothesis that predicts improvement with a phase advance. In either case, the statistically significant lower depression ratings after morning light compared with those after evening light provide strong support for the phase-shift hypothesis.

The following winter, 2 hours of morning bright light was compared with 0.5 hour, both beginning at 6 A.M. (Lewy et al. 1988). There were two baseline (adaptation or withdrawal) weeks. Although most patients who showed an obviously more robust antidepressant response to one light exposure over the other responded better to the 2-hour exposure, a few patients responded better to the 0.5-hour exposure. Perhaps these patients were becoming overly phase advanced with the longer light exposure.

When the patients completed the study, we asked them to reduce light exposure duration to determine the minimal amount necessary to maintain their euthymia. On average, patients were able to reduce the duration of morning light to 35.4 ± 5.1 (mean $\pm$ SE) minutes. In this study, there was a statistically significant relationship between the average DLMO and the mean depression rating for the five study conditions (prebaseline, adaptation week, withdrawal week, 0.5-hour morning-light week, and 2-hour morning-light week). The earlier the DLMO, the lower the depression rating (Figure 6-8).

Half of the patients in this study began with a baseline adaptation week. The other half began with a light-treatment week. Morning light was antidepressant if it was administered the 2nd week; however, it was not antidepressant if it was administered the 1st week. We have interpreted this "order" effect in the following way. We schedule sleep earlier for the entire study so that patients can awaken at 6 A.M. and finish the morning light treatment by 8 A.M. (so patients can go to work, etc.). We think that if sleep is advanced along with advancing the other rhythms, the phase angle between the endogenous circadian rhythms and sleep does not close within the 1st week, which will retard the antidepressant response. Perhaps sleep must be adapted to its new (earlier) phase position for a few days and the advance portion of the PRC must be "uncovered" (by advancing sleep) to achieve a maximal antidepressant response to morning bright light. This latter point may be relevant for recent studies in which morning light was scheduled whenever patients awakened and that did not find a maximal antidepressant response to morning light (C.I. Eastman, personal communication; M. Terman, personal communication).

During the winter of 1986–1987, the first morning- versus evening-light study was repeated, except that evening light was scheduled 1 hour earlier, DLMOs were obtained midweek and at the end of the week, and a 4th week was not done (Sack et al., in press). Evening light was scheduled 1 hour earlier because we thought that there was a slight chance that patients had not responded better to evening light in our first study due to a possible interference with sleep, which was scheduled to begin immediately after the evening light exposure.

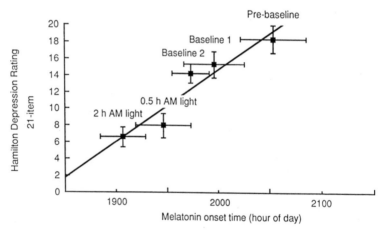

Figure 6-8. Correlation between melatonin onsets and Hamilton depression ratings in study of 0.5 hour versus 2 hours of light. Patients received either 0.5 or 2 hours of morning light immediately on awakening at 6 A.M. or woke into dim light during baseline weeks in a randomized crossover design. Five plotted points are as follows (from *left* to *right*): 1st day of the study, 1st baseline week, 2nd baseline week, week of 0.5 hour of morning light, and week of 2 hours of morning light. Linear regression, fitted for the five data points obtained for each of 12 subjects for whom we had completed data, showed significant correlation ($r = .95$, df 4, $P \leq .01$). When slopes were calculated for each subject individually, mean slope was also significantly different from 0 ($P \leq .006$, df 11, Student's t test). Data indicate that clinical improvement is highly correlated with phase advance in melatonin onset. Reprinted from Lewy et al. 1988, with permission from publisher.

Also, in our first study, because of the dim-light conditions in the evening required for the DLMO, patients received one more day of morning light treatment than of evening light treatment. Consequently, in this second study, patients were not exposed to morning bright light the day after a DLMO determination.

As in our first study, morning light advanced the DLMOs (more so in the patients than in the control subjects), and evening light delayed the DLMOs (more so in the control subjects than in the patients). Combining data from the second with the first morning-versus evening-light study, patients' DLMOs were relatively delayed compared with those of control subjects. This was not the case when the 0.5-hour morning-light study data were included; however, this study was not designed to assess baseline DLMOs.

Once again, morning light was significantly more antidepressant than evening light. However, depression ratings at the end of the week of evening light were slightly but statistically lower than those at the end of the baseline week. This was not the case in our first study, in which evening light was scheduled 1 hour later. We interpret these results to mean that morning light is most antidepressant because of a phase-advancing effect combined with a nonspecific (placebo?) effect that is a component of the light exposure no matter what time of day it is scheduled. If the light is scheduled sufficiently late, a phase-delay effect might to some extent counteract the placebo effect. If the light is scheduled in the early evening, there may be just the placebo effect, unopposed by any phase-delay effect.

There may be other ways that evening light is antidepressant in some patients. If sleep is not held constant and patients do not avoid bright light in the morning, evening light could energize patients, delay their sleep, and shift their wake-up time into the daylight, causing a phase advance of the DLMO relative to sleep (Lewy and Sack 1986). However, for most patients, morning light appears to be more antidepressant than evening light.

THE ADVANCE-DELAY DIFFERENTIAL AS A CIRCADIAN PHASE MARKER

If a patient has a winter depression of the rare phase-advance type, evening light might have a real therapeutic effect by providing a corrective phase delay. In fact, we have evidence for two such evening-light responders. One such patient had the most phase-advanced DLMO of any that we have ever measured. Interestingly, he was extremely hypersomnic in the winter, and his sleep onset appeared to cue to dusk throughout the year. If tested under the appropriate experimental conditions (i.e., temporal isolation), we would predict that he would have an intrinsic period shorter than 24 hours (which is extremely rare). Another clear-cut evening-light responder was in our first morning- versus evening-light study (Lewy et al. 1987a). Her 21-item Hamilton depression rating at the end of the week of morning light was 17 (Figure 6-6). At the end of the week of evening light, it was 4. Although her DLMO was quite early, it was not the earliest for that group of patients. However, she did have an advance-delay (A-D) differential that indicated that she was the most phase advanced of the patients studied that year.

The A-D differential is computed by determining a DLMO after the end of a week of baseline conditions, after a week of morning light, and after a week of evening light. The delay of the DLMO after the week of evening light (relative to baseline) is subtracted from the advance of the DLMO after the week of morning light (relative to baseline). For example, if a patient has a baseline DLMO of 2,100, a morning-light DLMO of 2,000, and an evening-light DLMO of 2,130, the A-D differential would be $1 - 0.5 = 0.5$ hours. We have hypothesized that the greater (or more positive) the A-D differential, the more phase delayed is the PRC. The one evening-light responder in our first study was the only patient with a negative A-D differential (her delay response to evening light was greater than her advance response to morning light), suggesting that she was the most phase advanced of the patients (Lewy et al. 1987b).

It may turn out that the A-D differential is a more reliable method of phase typing than the baseline DLMO, although the two are highly correlated (Figure 6-9), suggesting that the DLMO marks the phase of its PRC, which provides further validation for the use of the DLMO as a marker for the phase of its endogenous circadian pacemaker. In our first two morning- versus evening-light studies, the A-D differential more significantly ($P \le .001$) discriminated patients from control subjects than did the baseline DLMO ($P \le .01$). This is not surprising, because the A-D differential takes into account interindividual differences in light sensitivity and in melatonin synthesis (such as the biochemical lag time) that might affect the baseline DLMO. An analogy can be made that the A-D differential is to the baseline DLMO as the glucose tolerance test is to the fasting glucose level. The former is useful in diagnosing circadian rhythm disorders (phase typing), the latter is useful in diagnosing diabetes.

Phase Typing and the Phase-Angle Disturbance

All individuals who are phase advanced or phase delayed are necessarily chronobiologically ill. For that matter, not all patients who have sleep or mood disorders have chronobiologic disturbances. However, bright light should be therapeutic to the extent that a sleep or mood disorder has a chronobiologic component, providing it is scheduled at the correct time. In these cases, phase typing is important.

It may turn out, however, that patients cannot be phase typed with respect to a normal population. For example, most patients with winter depression may be phase delayed when they are ill compared with when they are euthymic (have normal mood), but may not necessarily be phase delayed with respect to a normal control population. If this is so, the phase-delay disturbance would be state dependent (Lewy et al. 1987b), not normative. Whether the phase-delay disturbance is normative or state dependent, there may be additional biological and/or psychological variables that predispose susceptible individuals to become depressed when they phase delay in the winter.

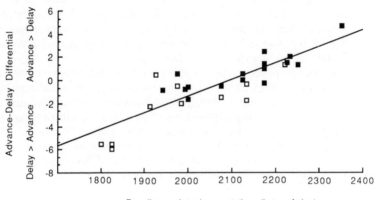

Baseline melatonin onset time (hour of day)

Figure 6-9. Baseline dim-light melatonin onset (DLMO) predicts advance-delay (A-D) differential. Melatonin onsets are determined in control subjects (□) and winter depressive patients (■) after 1 week of baseline conditions, after 1 week of morning bright light, and after 1 week of evening bright light. A-D differential is advance response to morning light minus delay response to evening light. Fitted regression line showed statistically significant ($P \leq .001$) correlation ($r = .86$), indicating that the later the baseline melatonin onset, the greater the A-D differential. This finding is consistent with the hypothesis that melatonin onset is marking the phase of its phase response curve, providing evidence that DLMO is a valid marker for phase of its endogenous circadian pacemaker. Reprinted from Lewy et al. 1988, with permission from publisher. Copyright 1988, Pergamon Press plc.

The phase-delay disturbance is therefore a necessary causal factor for most patients with winter depression; it is not yet known if it is a sufficient cause.

As mentioned earlier, there seems to be a phase-angle disturbance in winter depression, in that sleep is not as delayed as the other endogenous circadian rhythms (which are marked by the melatonin onset). In the four studies reported above, we held sleep constant while we advanced the other endogenous circadian rhythms with morning light, thus reducing the phase angle between sleep and these rhythms. We have also done two pilot studies, in which we delayed sleep while we held the phase of the endogenous circadian rhythms constant with midmorning light (Lewy et al. 1988, 1990). Delaying sleep under these conditions also appears to be an effective antidepressant for these patients (see Figures 6-10 through 6-12 for diagrams of these protocols). Perhaps society is partly the cause of winter depression, in that these patients are constrained to get up at the same time in the winter as in the summer; in the winter, sleep offset may occur before dawn, widening the phase angle between sleep offset and dawn.

In our most recent study, 2 weeks of light exposure were used and a withdrawal week separated the two (morning versus evening) light treatment conditions. Although the absence of these modifications in our previous studies would only bias the results against our hypothesis, we thought that these changes should be made. Otherwise, this study was similar in design to our second morning- versus evening-light study, except that DLMOs were determined only at the end of each week. The depression rating data from this study replicated the data from our first morning- versus evening-light study (Lewy et al. 1980). DLMO data have not yet been completed.

SUMMARY AND DISCUSSION

In summary, it is not known whether the phase-delay abnormality is the only predisposing factor for winter depression. However, it is likely that it is mediating the short-day stimulus that is causing the annual recurrence of winter depression in these patients. Apparently, patients with winter depression, cuing (as most humans do who have intrinsic circadian periods greater than 24 hours [Wever 1979]) to dawn more than to dusk, delay in the winter with the later dawn. Thus, winter depression—at least mechanistically—seems to be related more to a circadian rhythm disturbance than to seasonal rhythms. For most patients, the antidepressant response to bright light appears to be at least in part related to phase-advancing circadian rhythms with respect to real time and to sleep.

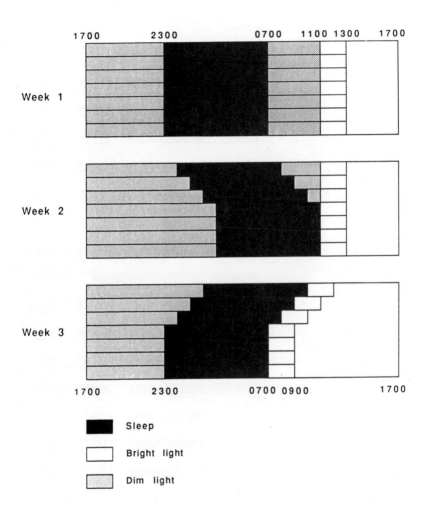

Figure 6-10. Protocol for our first shifted-sleep pilot study. Patients were admitted to clinical research center for 3-week period. During week 1, they were adapted to short day (dim light from 5 to 11 P.M.) and structured sleep schedule (11 P.M. to 7 A.M.). During week 2, sleep was gradually delayed so that by end of 2nd week, patients were awakening into bright light (total light exposure was kept constant). During week 3, sleep and morning light exposure were gradually advanced together. Patients gradually improved, beginning in middle of 2nd week.

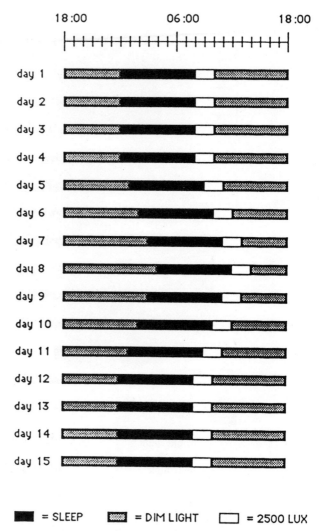

Figure 6-11. Protocol for "narrow phase angle" group of our second shifted-sleep pilot study. Sleep times were gradually delayed over 1st week and advanced back to baseline during 2nd week. Two hours of bright-light exposure were administered immediately on awakening at all points of study. For both groups of patients (see Figure 6-12), 2 hours of bright-light treatment was the only bright light received. At all other times, patients were kept in a dim room (<50 lux).

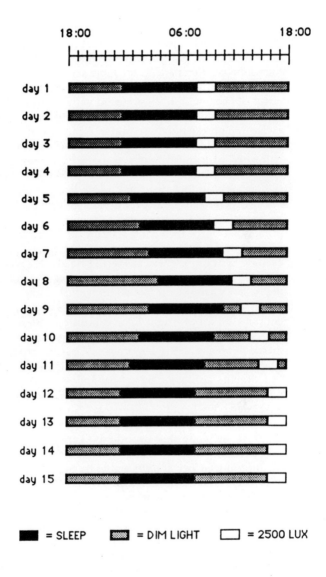

Figure 6-12. Protocol for "wide phase angle" group of our second shifted-sleep pilot study. For this group, 2-hour bright-light exposure was delayed, even as sleep times were advanced back to baseline, thus further widening phase angle between sleep and bright-light exposure.

What is causing the apparent phase delay in these patients? One possibility is that these patients are subsensitive to light; however, our preliminary data suggest that this does not seem to be the case. As mentioned earlier, patients are more sensitive to the phase-advancing effect of morning light but are less sensitive to the phase-delaying effect of evening light—compared with control subjects. According to results from an investigation still in progress on the suppression of melatonin production in response to 500 lux of light between 2 A.M. and 4 P.M., winter depressive patients may be more sensitive to light compared with control subjects, but we have not studied a sufficient number of patients to know if this difference will be statistically significant. Another, we think more likely, explanation is that the intrinsic periods of these patients are abnormally long. This needs to be tested under the appropriate experimental conditions (i.e., temporal isolation), which will hopefully be done in the near future.

There is no doubt that morning light causes phase advances and evening light causes phase delays. There also seems to be less and less doubt that morning light is a more effective treatment for winter depression than evening light. Individual studies that have failed to show superior efficacy for morning light did not hold sleep time constant or avoid bright-light exposure around twilight, which is critical when testing the phase-shift hypothesis or testing the relative merits of an alternative hypothesis. We have critiqued most of these studies elsewhere (Lewy and Sack 1986, 1988). The results from our experiments and from those that follow the same methodological guidelines for testing the phase-shift hypothesis (Avery et al. 1989) have been consistently confirmatory. Furthermore, despite the varied methodologies, the pooled analysis of all studies done to date also supports the phase-shift hypothesis (Terman et al. 1989).

We think it unlikely that an overall increase in light sensitivity in the morning (which at most would be two- or threefold, if one exists at all, even if there is no increased adaptation with the "brighter" light) would explain why patients become worse when switched to evening light, because, as mentioned earlier, patients frequently decrease their morning light exposure time by 75% (to 35.4 ± 5.1 [mean ± SE] minutes) to maintain the antidepressant response initiated by 2 hours of exposure to 2,500 lux of light. Furthermore, when patients are switched from 1 week of 2 hours of morning light to 1 week of 0.5 hour of morning light, they do not become statistically significantly more depressed (Lewy et al. 1988). Even with a withdrawal week between treatments, patients do as well on 0.5 hour as they do on 2 hours of morning light, provided that the 0.5-hour light treatment is the second treatment (Wirz-Justice et al. 1987). Moreover, patients who are clear-cut evening-light responders relapse when switched to morning light (Lewy et al. 1988), and hypothesizing a different circadian light-sensitivity rhythm for these patients (if it exists) still invokes different phase types for morning- and evening-light responders. An important question remains: Other than for the few phase-advanced patients, is evening light really effective in the treatment of winter depression, or is the response noted in some patients merely a nonspecific placebo effect?

Finally, it should be mentioned that another circadian rhythm hypothesis has been proposed which states that bright light is antidepressant by increasing the amplitude of the circadian pacemaker (Czeisler et al. 1987). This hypothesis is not mutually exclusive with the phase-shift hypothesis. Furthermore, recent preliminary data from our group and another group (D. Avery, personal communication) showed no difference in circadian amplitude between patients and control subjects and, more importantly, showed no increase in amplitude after patients responded to the antidepressant effect of bright light.

We are particularly interested in those few patients who preferentially respond to evening light; these patients may be responding to a corrective phase delay. If investigators think that evening light that is not capable of causing a phase advance is an ineffective antidepressant for the majority of winter depressive patients, we await further research to demonstrate that this is more than a nonspecific placebo effect.

REFERENCES

Arendt J: Melatonin assays in body fluids. J Neural Transm [Suppl] 13:265–278, 1978

Aschoff J (ed): Biological Rhythms. New York, Plenum, 1981a

Aschoff J: Annual rhythms in man, in Biological Rhythms. Edited by Aschoff J. New York, Plenum, 1981b

Avery D, Kahn A, Dager SR, et al: Bright light treatment of winter depression: AM compared to PM light (abstract). Biol Psychiatry 25:83A, 1989

Czeisler CA, Kronauer RE, Mooney JJ, et al: Biologic rhythm disorders, depression, and phototherapy: a new hypothesis. Psychiatr Clin North Am 10:687–709, 1987

Decoursey PJ: Function of a light rhythm in hamsters. Journal of Cellular and Comparative Physiology 63:189–196, 1964

Fiske VM, Bryant GK, Putnam J: Effect of light on the weight of the pineal in the rat. Endocrinology 66:489–491, 1960

Illnerová H, Vanecek J: Complex control of the circadian rhythm in N-acetyltransferase activity in the rat pineal gland, in Vertebrate Circadian Systems. Edited by Aschoff J, Daan S, Gross G. Berlin, Springer, 1982, pp 285–296

Illnerová H, Zvolsky P, Vanecek J: The circadian rhythm in plasma melatonin concentration of the urbanized man: the effect of summer and winter time. Brain Res 328:186–189, 1985

James SP, Wehr TA, Sack DA, et al: Treatment of seasonal affective disorder with evening light. Br J Psychiatry 147:424–428, 1985

Jimerson DC, Lynch HK, Post RM, et al: Urinary melatonin rhythms during sleep deprivation in depressed patients and normals. Life Sci 20:1501–1508, 1977

Kern HE, Lewy AJ: Corrections and additions to the history of light therapy and seasonal affective disorder. Arch Gen Psychiatry 47:90–91, 1990

Klein DC: Circadian rhythms in the pineal gland, in Endocrine Rhythms. Edited by Krieder DT. New York, Raven, 1979, pp 203–223

Klein DC, Weller JL: A rapid light-induced decrease in pineal serotonin N-acetyltransferase activity. Science 177:532–533, 1972

Kripke DF: Photoperiodic mechanisms for depression and its treatment, in Biological Psychiatry. Edited by Perris C, Struwe G, Jansson B. Amsterdam, Elsevier, 1981, pp 1249–1252

Kripke DF: Critical interval hypotheses for depression. Chronobiol Int 1:73–80, 1984

Kripke DF, Mullaney DJ, Atkinson ML, et al: Circadian rhythm disorders in manic-depressives. Biol Psychiatry 13:335–351, 1978

Kripke DF, Mullaney DS, Savides TJ, et al: Phototherapy for nonseasonal major depressive disorders, in Seasonal Affective Disorders and Phototherapy. Edited by Rosenthal NE, Blehar MC. New York, Guilford, 1989, pp 342–356

Lewy AJ: Biochemistry and regulation of mammalian melatonin production, in The Pineal Gland. Edited by Relkin RM. New York, Elsevier North-Holland, 1983, pp 77–128

Lewy AJ, Markey SP: Analysis of melatonin in human plasma gas chromatography negative chemical ionization mass spectrometry. Science 201:741–743, 1978

Lewy AJ, Sack RL: Minireview: light therapy and psychiatry. Proc Soc Exp Biol Med 183:11–18, 1986

Lewy AJ, Sack RL: The phase-shift hypothesis of seasonal affective disorder. Am J Psychiatry 145:1041–1042, 1988

Lewy AJ, Wehr TA, Goodwin FK, et al: Light suppresses melatonin secretion in humans. Science 210:1267–1269, 1980

Lewy AJ, Kern HE, Rosenthal NE, et al: Bright artificial light treatment of a manic-depressive patient with a seasonal mood cycle. Am J Psychiatry 139:1496–1498, 1982

Lewy AJ, Sack RL, Fredrickson RH, et al: The use of bright light in the treatment of chronobiologic sleep and mood disorders: the phase-response curve. Psychopharmacol Bull 19:523–525, 1983

Lewy AJ, Sack RL, Singer CM: Assessment and treatment of chronobiologic disorders using plasma melatonin levels and bright light exposure: the clock-gate model and the phase response curve. Psychopharmacol Bull 20:561–565, 1984

Lewy AJ, Sack RL, Singer CM: Immediate and delayed effects of bright light on human melatonin production: shifting "dawn" and "dusk" shifts the dim light melatonin onset (DLMO). Ann NY Acad Sci 452:253–259, 1985a

Lewy AJ, Sack RL, Singer CM: Treating phase typed chronobiologic sleep and mood disorders using appropriately timed bright artificial light. Psychopharmacol Bull 21:368–372, 1985b

Lewy AJ, Sack RL, Singer CM: Melatonin, light and chronobiological disorders, in Photoperiodism, Melatonin and the Pineal. Edited by Evered D, Clark S. New York, Pergamon, 1985c, pp 231–252

Lewy AJ, Nurnberger JI, Wehr TA, et al: Supersensitivity to light: possible trait marker for manic-depressive illness. Am J Psychiatry 142:725–727, 1985d

Lewy AJ, Sack RL, Miller LS, et al: Antidepressant and circadian phase-shifting effects of light. Science 235:352–354, 1987a

Lewy AJ, Sack RL, Singer CM, et al: The phase shift hypothesis for bright light's therapeutic mechanism of action: theoretical considerations and experimental evidence. Psychopharmacol Bull 23:349–353, 1987b

Lewy AJ, Sack RL, Singer CM, et al: Winter depression and the phase shift hypothesis for bright light's therapeutic effects: history, theory and experimental evidence. Journal of Biological Rhythms 3:121–134, 1988

Lewy AJ, Sack RL, Singer CM, et al: Winter depression: the phase angle between sleep and other circadian rhythms may be critical, in Seasonal Affective Disorder. Edited by Thompson C, Silverstone T. London, Clinical Neuroscience Publishers, 1990, pp 211–228

Lynch HJ, Jimerson DC, Ozaki Y, et al: Entrainment of rhythmic melatonin secretion in man to a 12-hour phase shift in the light dark cycle. Life Sci 23:1557–1564, 1977

Mueller PD, Allen NG: Diagnosis and treatment of severe light-sensitive seasonal energy syndrome (SES) and its relationship to melatonin anabolism. Fair Oaks Hospital Psychiatry Letter 2(9), 1984

Papousek M: Chronobiological aspects of cyclothymia. Fortschr Neurol Psychiatr 43:381–440, 1975

Pittendrigh CS, Daan S: A functional analysis of circadian pacemakers in nocturnal rodents, IV: entrainment: pacemaker as clock. J Comp Physiol [A] 106:291–331, 1976

Quay WB: Circadian and estrus rhythms in pineal melatonin and 5-hydroxyindole-3-acetic acid. Proc Soc Exp Biol Med 115:710–713, 1964

Reiter RJ, Hurlbut EC, Brainard GC, et al: Influence of light irradiance on hydroxyindole-O-methyltransferase activity, serotonin-N-acetyl-transferase activity, and radioimmunoassayable melatonin levels in the pineal gland of the diurnally active Richardson's ground squirrel. Brain Res 288:151–157, 1983

Rosenthal NE, Lewy AJ, Wehr TA, et al: Seasonal cycling in a bipolar patient. Psychiatr Res 8:25–31, 1983

Rosenthal NE, Sack DA, Gillin JC, et al: Seasonal affective disorder. Arch Gen Psychiatry 41:72–80, 1984

Rosenthal NE, Sack DA, Carpenter CD, et al: Antidepressant effects of light in seasonal affective disorder. Am J Psychiatry 142:163–170, 1985

Sack RL, Lewy AJ, White DM, et al: Morning versus evening light treatment for winter depression: evidence that the therapeutic effects of light are mediated by circadian phase shifts. Arch Gen Psychiatry (in press)

Terman M, Terman JS, Quitkin FM, et al: Light therapy for seasonal affective disorder. Neuropsychopharmacology 2:1–22, 1989

Vaughan GM, Bell R, De La Pena A: Nocturnal plasma melatonin in humans: episodic pattern and influence of light. Neuroscience Letters 14:81–84, 1979

Wehr TA, Rosenthal NE: In reply. Arch Gen Psychiatry 46:194–195, 1989

Wehr TA, Wirz-Justice A, Goodwin FK, et al: Phase advance of the circadian sleep-wake cycle as an antidepressant. Science 206:710–713, 1979

Wehr TA, Jacobsen FM, Sack DA, et al: Phototherapy of seasonal affective disorder: time of day and suppression of melatonin are not critical for antidepressant effects. Arch Gen Psychiatry 43:870–875, 1986

Weitzman ED, Weinberg U, D'Eletto R, et al: Studies of the 24 hour rhythm of melatonin in man. J Neural Transm [Suppl] 13:265–278, 1978

Wetterberg L: Melatonin in humans: physiological and clinical studies. J Neural Transm [Suppl] 13:289–310, 1978

Wever RA (ed): The Circadian System of Man. New York, Springer-Verlag, 1979

Wever RA, Polasek J, Wildgruber C: Bright light affects human circadian rhythms. Pflugers Arch 396:85–87, 1983

Wirz-Justice A, Schmid AC, Graw P, et al: Dose relationships of morning bright white light in seasonal affective disorders (SAD). Experientia 43:574–576, 1987

Wurtman RJ, Axelrod J, Phillips LS: Melatonin synthesis in the pineal gland: control by light. Science 142:1071–1073, 1963

Zucker I: Seasonal affective disorders: animal models. Journal of Biological Rhythms 3:209–223, 1988

Chapter 7

Melatonin, Light Therapy, and Premenstrual Syndrome

Barbara L. Parry, M.D.
Sarah L. Berga, M.D.
Daniel F. Kripke, M.D.
J.C. Gillin, M.D.

Chapter 7

Melatonin, Light Therapy, and Premenstrual Syndrome

Premenstrual syndrome (PMS), currently termed late luteal phase dysphoric disorder (LLPDD) in DSM-III-R (American Psychiatric Association 1987), is a disorder in which mood and behavior disturbances occur during the late luteal phase of the menstrual cycle and remit shortly after the onset of menses. Reproductive and behavior changes occur in certain animal species in association not only with the ovarian cycle but also in response to the changing seasons. These seasonal changes are thought to be mediated by the hormone melatonin, which is secreted from the pineal gland in response to the environmental light-dark cycle (Tamarkin et al. 1985). Melatonin also may mediate changes in mood and behavior in patients with seasonal PMS whose depressive symptoms occur during the premenstrual phase in the fall and winter and remit in the spring and summer in association with changes in the light-dark cycle (Parry et al. 1987). Whether melatonin mediates the cyclic changes in mood and behavior occurring in association with the menstrual cycle in women with nonseasonal PMS will be the focus of the first part of this chapter. The studies investigating melatonin and the menstrual cycle and melatonin and depression will be reviewed as background material for presenting the rationale, experimental design, and results of a study of melatonin in nonseasonal-PMS patients. In the second part of this chapter, we will discuss the effects of bright-light therapy in PMS patients and how these effects may be mediated by and reflected in changes of the melatonin circadian rhythm.

MELATONIN AND THE MENSTRUAL CYCLE

The studies of melatonin during the human menstrual cycle often have not measured the circadian profile of melatonin secretion or have not examined melatonin in relation to mood and behavior changes. Hariharasubramanian et al. (1984) examined the circadian rhythm of plasma melatonin during different phases of the normal human menstrual cycle and found a phase delay of the nocturnal peak of melatonin during the midmenstrual period (midcycle). In another study of circadian melatonin secretion, a delay in the onset of melatonin secretion in the luteal phase compared with the follicular phase of the menstrual cycle was found in a patient with seasonal PMS (Parry et al. 1987). Webley and Leidenberger (1986) measured serum melatonin every 4 hours, from which they derived a melatonin index. An increased melatonin index was associated with an increase in the dose of progestin in eight women taking a three-phase contraceptive pill. In women with normal menstrual cycles, Brzezinski et al. (1988) measured melatonin every 2 hours and Berga and Yen (1988) every 30 minutes during the night over a 24-hour period and found no change in melatonin with menstrual cycle phase.

In urine studies of melatonin secretion, Penny (1982) found that follicular phase excretion was significantly greater than luteal phase excretion. Fellenberg et al. (1982) measured the excretion of 6-sulphatoxymelatonin and found that the amount of melatonin excreted per day remained relatively constant throughout the menstrual cycle. Hamilton et al. (1988), measuring daily 24-hour urinary 6-hydroxymelatonin, found relatively stable levels during the menstrual cycle in women reporting premenstrual dysphoria.

In noncircadian studies, Wetterberg et al. (1976) measured serum melatonin in the morning at 2- to 3-day intervals in five healthy women and showed that melatonin was elevated at the time of menstrual bleeding and had its nadir at the time of ovulation. Wirz-Justice and Arendt (1979) measured plasma melatonin daily at 8 A.M. during the menstrual cycle and also found a nadir occurring just before the luteinizing hormone (LH) surge and ovulation with peaks occurring in the mid follicular phase (cycle day 8) and late luteal phase (cycle day 26).

MELATONIN AND DEPRESSION

Increasing evidence suggests a relationship between premenstrual syndrome and major depressive disorders (Halbreich and Endicott 1985; Hallman 1986; Mackenzie et al. 1986; Schuckit et al. 1975; Wetzel et al. 1975). Many women with PMS later develop mood disorders (Schukit et al. 1975; Wetzel et al. 1975) and a majority of women with premenstrual depression have a lifelong history of major depressive disorder (Halbreich and Endicott 1985).

Some, but not all, studies have found abnormally low levels of melatonin secretion in depression (Beck-Friis et al. 1984; Brown et al. 1985; Claustrat et al. 1984; Lewy et al. 1979; Mendlewicz et al. 1979; Thompson et al. 1988; Wetterberg et al. 1982). Thus, given the relationship of PMS and mood disorders, one might hypothesize that low levels of melatonin might also be found in patients with PMS, similar to the findings in some groups of depressed patients.

MELATONIN AS A MEASURE OF CIRCADIAN RHYTHM DISTURBANCES

Some investigators have hypothesized that in depression the oscillator regulating the circadian rhythms of rapid eye movement (REM) sleep, temperature, cortisol, and melatonin is shifted earlier (phase advanced) with respect to the sleep-wake cycle (Kripke et al. 1978; Wehr and Goodwin 1980). Given the relationship of PMS and depressive disorders, one could hypothesize a similar phase-advance disturbance in PMS. A phase-advance hypothesis of PMS is supported by several theoretical and empirical observations. First, estrogen advances and progesterone delays circadian rhythms in animals (Albers et al. 1981). If these hormones have similar circadian effects in humans, progesterone deficiency, postulated in PMS (Abraham et al. 1978; Backstrom and Carstensen 1974; Backstrom et al. 1976; Munday et al. 1981), theoretically should produce phase-advance disturbances, because not enough progesterone would be available to antagonize the phase-advancing properties of estrogen. Second, our preliminary sleep and temperature studies in PMS patients suggest phase-advance abnormalities (Parry and Wehr 1987; Parry et al., in press). In PMS patients, melatonin could be used to measure circadian phase and thereby test whether circadian rhythms are abnormally advanced, as they are in some patients with major depression. Therefore, to investigate a phase-advance hypothesis of PMS, we measured circadian phase with melatonin, a hormone that is reported to be less sensitive than cortisol to the masking effects of sleep, locomotor activity, and stress (Lewy et al. 1985).

MELATONIN AND PMS

We measured melatonin in PMS patients to determine whether

1. Changes in melatonin secretion occur in association with mood and behavior changes in PMS patients during different hormonal phases of the menstrual cycle
2. Abnormally low levels of melatonin occur in patients with premenstrual depression similar to that reported in patients with major depression

3. Circadian phase disturbances as measured by melatonin occur in PMS patients as in some patients with other recurrent depressive disorders.

Experimental Design

Subjects. The patients were referred by local professionals or were recruited by advertisement. Screening procedures consisted of a structured questionnaire and psychiatric interview, physical examination, and laboratory tests, including chemistry panel, complete blood count, urinalysis, and measurement of thyroid indices. If the patient had no history of major medical, gynecologic, or psychiatric illness, had regular (26- to 32-day) menstrual cycles, appeared to have premenstrual symptoms sufficiently severe to disrupt social or occupational functioning, and was willing to endure the rigors of a long-term research study, she was entered into a 2- to 3-month diagnostic evaluation.

During the evaluation, patients completed twice-daily mood ratings (100-mm line-segmented scales for depression, anxiety, irritability, fatigue, withdrawal, and global sense of well-being) and visited the clinic weekly for standardized observer (21-item Hamilton Rating Scale for Depression [HAM-D]; Hamilton 1960) and subjective (Beck Depression Inventory [BDI]; Beck et al. 1961) depression ratings. To be selected for the study, patients had to meet DSM-III-R criteria for LLPDD, have mean scores ≥14 on the HAM-D and ≥10 on the BDI premenstrually (the week preceding the onset of menses), and demonstrate a reduction of scores to ≤7 on the HAM-D and ≤5 on the BDI by the week after cessation of menses. To be included, the subject's mean daily depression ratings during the luteal phase also had to be 30% greater than those during the follicular phase. Also, patients could not have been on birth control pills for at least 6 months before the study and had to agree to use no medication or drugs (including alcohol) for at least 1 month before initiating the study. Control subjects, matched for age and cycle phase, were without reported premenstrual mood disorders.

The protocol was approved by the University of California, San Diego (UCSD), Human Subjects Committee. All subjects gave written informed consent after the nature and possible consequences of the studies had been fully explained.

Methods. Overnight hormonal sampling was done in patients at each of four different menstrual cycle phases: mid follicular (cycle day [CD] 8 ± 2 after menses), late follicular (CD 12 ± 2), midluteal (7 ± 2 days after the LH surge), and late luteal (12 ± 2 days after the LH surge).

The midcycle LH surge was determined by a colorimetric urinary immunoassay (Ovustick, Irvine, California). Subjects were admitted to the general clinical research center of the UCSD Medical Center at 5 P.M. An indwelling intravenous catheter was inserted, and samples for melatonin determination were drawn every 30 minutes from 6 P.M. to 9 A.M. So as not to disturb sleep, samples after 11 P.M. were obtained from an intravenous line connected to an adjoining room through a porthole. Patients were kept in dim-light (< 100 lux) conditions between 6 and 11 P.M., asked to sleep in a dark room from 11 P.M. to 7 A.M., and then kept in dim light again from 7 to 9 A.M. Baseline levels for estradiol and progesterone were drawn at 6 P.M. at each admission. Control subjects were studied at similar times under similar conditions. The cycle phase of control subjects was estimated from the day of the LH surge as determined by daily serum LH measurements.

Hormone assays. Plasma samples for melatonin were collected in ethylenediaminetetraacetic acid (EDTA)–containing plastic tubes and centrifuged, and the plasma was frozen immediately and stored at −20°C until assay. Plasma melatonin was measured directly, without extraction, by a previously described radioimmunoassay (RIA) (Berga et al. 1988). The accuracy of the RIA was validated by gas chromatography–mass spectroscopy methods (Lewy and Markey 1978). Assay sensitivity was 43 pmol/L (10 pg/ml). Samples were analyzed in duplicate. Selected samples from control subjects and PMS patients were run in the same assay. The intra- and interassay coefficients of variation were 6.5 and 8.7%, respectively.

The concentrations of serum estradiol and progesterone were determined by RIAs (Anderson et al. 1976; Lasley et al. 1975).

Data analyses. Melatonin secretion was analyzed for onset and offset time, midpoint, peak, duration, and area under the curve (AUC) with the following criteria: The onset of melatonin secretion was defined as the time of the first point that was detectable (>10 pg/ml) or exceeded the mean baseline levels between 6 and 8 P.M. and also was followed by two consecutive points of equal or lesser magnitude. The offset time was defined as the time at which the melatonin level was nondetectable or fell below mean baseline levels and also was followed by two consecutive points of equal or lesser magnitude. The peak of melatonin was determined by both the single highest point between 11 P.M. and 6 A.M. and the mean of the three highest points between 11 P.M. and 6 A.M. However, as similar results were obtained by both methods, only the data with the single highest point to define the peak are presented. AUC was determined by the integrated melatonin level from 6 P.M. to 9 A.M. Duration was defined as the time between onset and offset. The midpoint was defined as the time midway between onset and offset.

Some women, both control subjects and PMS patients, did not demonstrate a melatonin rise at various menstrual cycle phases. In these cases, melatonin onset, offset, and midpoint could not be derived. To account for "empty cells" in these cases, a mixed factor analysis of variance (ANOVA) with repeated measures (NCSS, Kaysville, Utah) was used to determine group (PMS versus control) effects, menstrual cycle phase (early follicular, late follicular, mid luteal, and late luteal) effects, and interaction. Post hoc t tests with Bonferonni correction were applied to identify specific menstrual cycle phase differences when there were significant main effects by ANOVA.

For arithmetic purposes, clock hours were converted to a 360° 24-hour clock with 2400 equal to 360°. A P value of $\leq.05$ was considered statistically significant.

Results

Patient demographics. Eight of 40 patients who were screened were selected for the study. Reasons for exclusion included irregular menstrual cycles, being on oral contraceptives or other medication, and not meeting diagnostic criteria for LLPDD. The mean age of both PMS patients and control subjects was 30 years (range 26–34). There were no significant differences between control subjects and PMS patients for age, height, or weight, and significant melatonin parameters and season of the year studied did not correlate. The PMS patients generally reported suffering from their disorder for more than 5 years.

Reproductive hormone analyses. Measurements made during the mid follicular phase by historical data were actually made during the early follicular phase by endocrine data; thus the latter term was used in subsequent analyses to reflect menstrual cycle phase more accurately. With a mixed two-factor ANOVA, there were significant menstrual cycle phase effects for serum estradiol and progesterone: both PMS patients and control subjects displayed the expected elevations in serum estradiol during the late follicular and mid luteal phases, as well as the expected elevation of progesterone during the mid luteal phase. There were no significant differences between groups (PMS versus control) for serum estradiol or progesterone levels.

Melatonin analyses. To examine overall differences in the PMS versus the control group, each of the melatonin parameters previously described (melatonin onset, midpoint, offset, peak, duration, and

AUC) were analyzed for menstrual cycle phase differences for each group separately, and then the groups were compared by group *t* test.

Melatonin parameters did not differ according to menstrual cycle phase in either the PMS patients or control subjects when analyzed separately by a repeated-measures ANOVA (Berga and Yen 1988). When the groups were compared, women with PMS had an earlier offset of melatonin secretion. Onset time did not differ significantly between the two groups. In addition, a multivariate analysis showed that AUC and duration of melatonin secretion were lower in PMS patients than in control subjects, but melatonin peak was not significantly different between the two groups.

To examine phase differences between groups, a mixed two-factor ANOVA was used to determine main effects for groups (PMS versus control) and menstrual cycle phase (early follicular, late follicular, mid luteal, late luteal) for each of the melatonin parameters. In this analysis, PMS patients showed an earlier offset of melatonin secretion in the luteal phase.

In summary, significant differences were found in PMS patients versus control subjects for AUC, duration, and offset of melatonin secretion. The offset of melatonin secretion was most advanced in PMS patients compared with control subjects in the luteal phase, when PMS patients were most symptomatic. By visual inspection of the data, the mean level of melatonin secretion (as reflected in AUC) most closely approached that of control subjects during the late follicular phase when the mood of PMS patients also most closely approached that of control subjects. Thus, the overall waveform of melatonin secretion appeared different for PMS patients versus control subjects.

LIGHT THERAPY AND PMS

Because the timing (offset) of melatonin secretion was different in PMS patients compared with control subjects, we sought to correct this timing (phase) disturbance with bright-light therapy. Bright light in the morning advances circadian rhythms, and bright light in the evening delays circadian rhythms (Lewy et al. 1987; also see Chapter 6, this volume). Thus, bright light administered in the evening to PMS patients, who demonstrate earlier (phase-advanced) disturbances in melatonin circadian rhythms, would be expected to delay and thereby correct these circadian disturbances and result in improved mood. Alternatively, administration of bright morning light would be expected to exacerbate the phase-advance disturbances and thereby worsen mood. Thus, we used light therapy to test our hypothesis of phase-advance disturbances in PMS and to determine if, by correcting these underlying phase disturbances, we could induce clinical remission.

Experimental Design

Six PMS patients, selected with the aforementioned criteria, were randomized for 2 months to a crossover trial of morning (6:30–8:30 A.M.) versus evening (7–9 P.M.) bright-light treatment administered for 7 consecutive days during the symptomatic luteal phase of the menstrual cycle (7–10 days before the onset of menses). Patients were asked to sit 3 feet from a 2,500-lux light source (eight 40-watt VitaLite fluorescent bulbs, or a portable illumination box from Apollo Light, Orem, Utah), keep their eyes open, and gaze every few minutes at the light. During the month of the study, patients were asked to sleep from 10:30 P.M. to 6:30 A.M., to take no naps, and to document their sleep times and light exposure on daily sleep and light logs. They were also asked to wear goggles to block out high-intensity light exposure during morning hours when they received the evening light treatment and during the evening hours when they received the morning light treatment. This aspect of the study was designed to balance the amount of light exposure on both treatment conditions.

At the end of 7 days of light treatment in the luteal phase, two raters blind to the treatment condition assessed mood over the last several days with the HAM-D; an addendum to the HAM-D that assessed atypical depressive symptoms such as fatigue, social withdrawal, carbohydrate craving, weight gain, and hypersomnia (maximum 23 points); and a mania rating scale (N.E. Rosenthal and T.A. Wehr, unpublished data). The criterion of Terman et al. (1989) were used to determine the response to light treatment: a 50% reduction on the 21-item HAM-D to a score of < 8. In addition, after each treatment, the patients completed the BDI.

One patient did not complete the morning light treatment because of her spouse's objection. One patient who developed severe agitation after 2 days on 2 hours of morning light used only 1 hour of morning light the remainder of the week.

Results

By ANOVA, there were significant treatment effects for HAM-D ratings ($F = 16.10$, df 2,9; $P < .001$). BDI ratings approached significance ($F = 3.25$, df 2,8; $P \leq .09$). Post hoc t tests revealed that compared with baseline (the mean ratings obtained during the late luteal phase in the months before light treatment), there were significant reductions in HAM-D (t = 9.09, df 5; P < .003) and BDI (t = 3.87, df 4; P < .01) depression ratings after evening light treatment. After morning light treatment, there were no statistically significant differences from baseline in HAM-D (t = .63, df 4; NS) or BDI (t = 1.25, df 4; NS) ratings.

The differences between morning versus evening light on HAM-D (t = 1.49, df 4; NS) or BDI (t = 1.4, df 4; NS) depression ratings did not reach statistical significance. Also, delta (change) scores from baseline were not statistically significant between morning and evening light treatments. Mania scores were low throughout the study and, like the atypical depression ratings, did not vary significantly.

CONCLUSION

Compared with control subjects, PMS patients had an earlier offset time of melatonin secretion, which was most pronounced in the luteal phase. These findings suggest that PMS patients have a phase-advance disturbance of the circadian oscillator regulating melatonin secretion, which responds to treatment with bright evening light.

The relationship of PMS to circadian physiology also is supported by the fact that PMS patients respond to total and partial sleep deprivation, as do patients with major depressive disorder and in contrast to patients with panic disorder and obsessive-compulsive disorder (Gillin 1983; Joffe and Swinson 1988; Parry and Wehr 1987; Roy-Byrne et al. 1986). A phase-advance disturbance of circadian rhythms relative to the sleep-wake cycle should be correctable by either 1) delaying the advanced circadian rhythm or 2) advancing sleep. Clinical findings suggest that these interventions are effective in reducing symptoms in PMS patients. PMS patients preferentially respond to evening light, which delays circadian rhythms, compared with morning light, which advances these rhythms (Parry et al. 1989). Also, PMS patients improve more by advancing sleep (late-night partial sleep deprivation) than by delaying sleep (early-night partial sleep deprivation) (Parry and Wehr 1987).

Although the response to evening light is consistent with the hypothesis of a phase advance of circadian rhythms in this disorder, the benefits of morning light, although not significant, showed a favorable trend. That morning light did not exacerbate symptoms and was not significantly different from evening light suggests that the effects of light may not be mediated entirely through shifting circadian phase (Czeisler et al. 1987) and that, in this disorder, morning light cannot serve as an internal control. Our preliminary data suggest that morning light may increase the amplitude of melatonin secretion.

This finding suggests that morning light may exert its antidepressant effects by increasing the abnormally low levels of melatonin found in PMS patients.

Further trials with a larger number of patients and with an additional placebo control condition are warranted. Nonetheless, these initial results are promising and suggest that bright light may serve as an alternative to the pharmacologic management of PMS.

In summary, these data demonstrate that women with PMS manifest chronobiological abnormalities of melatonin secretion. The fact that the symptoms of such patients respond to specific treatments that affect circadian physiology, such as late-night sleep deprivation and evening bright light, suggests that circadian system abnormalities may contribute to the pathogenesis of PMS and that correcting such disturbances may result in clinical remission.

REFERENCES

Abraham GE, Elsner CW, Lucas LA: Hormonal and behavioral changes during the menstrual cycle. Senologia 3:33–38, 1978

Albers HE, Gerall AA, Axelson JF: Effect of reproductive state on circadian periodicity in the rat. Physiol Behav 26:21–25, 1981

American Psychiatric Association: Diagnostic and Statistical Manual of Mental Disorders, 3rd Edition, Revised. Washington, DC, American Psychiatric Association, 1987

Anderson DC, Hopper BR, Lasley BL, et al: A simple method for the assay of eight steroids in small volumes of plasma. Steriods 28:179–196, 1976

Backstrom T, Carstensen H: Estrogen and progesterone in plasma in relation to premenstrual tension. J Steroid Biochem 5:257–260, 1974

Backstrom T, Wide L, Soderga R, et al: FSH, LG, TeBG-capacity, estrogen and progesterone in women with premenstrual tension during the luteal phase. J Steroid Biochem 7:473–476, 1976

Beck AT, Ward CM, Mendelson M, et al: An inventory for measuring depression. Arch Gen Psychiatry 4:561–571, 1961

Beck-Friis J, Von Rosen D, Kjellman BF, et al: Melatonin in relation to body measures, sex, age, season and the use of drugs in patients with major affective disorder and healthy subjects. Psychoneuroendocrinology 9:261–277, 1984

Berga SL, Yen SSC: The human circadian pattern of plasma melatonin (MLT) during different menstrual cycle phases. Abstract presented at the 70th annual meeting of the Endocrine Society, New Orleans, LA, 1988

Berga SL, Mortola JF, Yen SSC: Amplication of nocturnal melatonin secretion in women with functional hypothalamic amenorrhea. J Clin Endocrinol Metab 66:242–244, 1988

Brown RP, Kocsis JH, Caroff S, et al: Differences in nocturnal melatonin secretion between melancholic depressed patients and control subjects. Am J Psychiatry 142:811–816, 1985

Brzezinski A, Lynch HJ, Seibel MM, et al: The circadian rhythm of plasma melatonin during the normal menstrual cycle and in amenorrheic women. J Clin Endocrinol Metab 66:891–895, 1988

Claustrat B, Chazot G, Brun J, et al: A chronobiological study of melatonin and cortisol secretion in depressed subjects: plasma melatonin, a biochemical marker in major depression. Biol Psychiatry 19:1215–1228, 1984

Czeisler CA, Kronauer RE, Mooney JJ, et al: Biologic rhythm disorders, depression and phototherapy: a new hypothesis, in Psychiatric Clinics of North America. Edited by Erman MK. Philadelphia, PA, WB Saunders, 1987, pp 687–709

Fellenberg AJ, Phillipou G, Seamark RF: Urinary 6 sulphatoxy melatonin excretion during the human menstrual cycle. Clin Endocrinol 17:71–75, 1982

Gillin JC: The sleep therapies of depression. Prog Neuropsychopharmacol Biol Psychiatry 7:351–364, 1983

Halbreich U, Endicott J: Relationship of dysphoric premenstrual changes to depressive disorders. Acta Psychiatr Scand 71:331–338, 1985

Hallman J: The premenstrual syndrome—an equivalent of depression? Acta Psychiatr Scand 73:403–411, 1986

Hamilton AA, Gallant SA, Pinkel S: Urinary 6-hydroxymelatonin in menstruating women. Biol Psychiatry 24:845–852, 1988

Hamilton M: A rating scale for depression. J Neurol Neurosurg Psychiatry 23:56–62, 1960

Hariharasubramanian N, Nair NPV, Pilapil C: Circadian rhythm of plasma melatonin and cortisol during the menstrual cycle, in The Pineal Gland: Endocrine Aspects. Edited by Brown GM, Wainwright SD. Oxford, Pergamon, 1984, pp 31–36

Joffe RT, Swinson RP: Total sleep deprivation in patients with obsessive-compulsive disorder. Acta Psychiatr Scand 77:483–487, 1988

Kripke DF, Mullaney DJ, Atkinson M, et al: Circadian rhythm disorders in manic depressives. Biol Psychiatry 13:335–351, 1978

Lasley BL, Wang CF, Yen SSC: The effects of estrogen and progesterone on the functional capacity of the gonadotrophs. J Clin Endocrinol Metab 42:820–826, 1975

Lewy AJ, Markey SP: Analysis of melatonin in human plasma by gas chromatography negative chemical ionization mass spectroscopy. Science 201:741–743, 1978

Lewy AJ, Wehr TA, Gold P, et al: Plasma melatonin in manic-depressive illness, in Catecholamines: Basic and Clinical Frontiers, Vol 2. Edited by Usdin E, Kopin IJ, Barchas J. New York, Pergamon, 1979, pp 1173–1175

Lewy AJ, Sack RL, Singer CM: Assessment and treatment of chronobiologic disorders using plasma melatonin levels and bright light exposure: the clock-gate model and the phase response curve. Psychopharm Academy Bulletin 20:561–565, 1984

Lewy AJ, Sack RL, Miller S, et al: Antidepressant and circadian phase-shifting effects of light. Science 235:352–354, 1987

Mackenzie TB, Wilcox K, Baron H: Lifetime prevalence of psychiatric disorders. J Affective Disord 10:15–19, 1986

Mendlewicz J, Linkowski P, Branchey L, et al: Abnormal 24-hour pattern of melatonin secretion in depression. Lancet 2:1362, 1979

Munday MR, Brush MG, Taylor RW: Correlations between progesterone, oestradiol and aldosterone levels in the premenstrual syndrome. Clin Endocrinol 14:1–9, 1981

Parry BL, Wehr TA: Therapeutic effect of sleep deprivation in patients with premenstrual syndrome. Am J Psychiatry 144:808–810, 1987

Parry BL, Rosenthal NE, Tamarkin L, et al: Treatment of a patient with seasonal premenstrual syndrome. Am J Psychiatry 144:762–766, 1987

Parry BL, Berga SL, Mostofi N, et al: Morning versus evening bright light treatment of late luteal phase dysphoric disorder. Am J Psychiatry 146:1215–1217, 1989

Parry BL, Mendelson WB, Sack DA, et al: Longitudinal sleep EEG, temperature and activity measurements across the menstrual cycle in patients with premenstrual depression and in age-matched controls. Psychiatry Res (in press)

Penny R: Melatonin excretion in normal males and females: increase during puberty. Metabolism 31:816–823, 1982

Roy-Byrne PP, Uhde TW, Post RM: Effects of one night's sleep deprivation on mood and behavior in panic disorder. Arch Gen Psychiatry 43:895–899, 1986

Schuckit MA, Daly V, Herman G, et al: Premenstrual symptoms and depression in a university population. Diseases of the Nervous System 36:516–517, 1975

Tamarkin L, Baird CJ, Almeida OFX: Melatonin: a coordinating signal for mammalian reproduction? Science 227:714–720, 1985

Terman M, Terman JS, Quitkin FM, et al: Light therapy for seasonal affective disorder: a review of efficacy. Neuropsychopharmacology 2:1–32, 1989

Thompson C, Franey C, Arendt J, et al: A comparison of melatonin secretion in depressed patients and normal subjects. Br J Psychiatry 152:260–265, 1988

Webley GE, Leidenberger F: The circadian pattern of melatonin and its positive relationship with progesterone in women. J Clin Endocrinol Metab 63:323–328, 1986

Wehr TA, Goodwin FK: Circadian rhythm desynchronization as a basis for manic-depressive cycles. Psychopharmacol Bull 16:19–20, 1980

Wetterberg L, Arendt J, Paunier L, et al: Human serum melatonin changes during the menstrual cycle. J Clin Endocrinol Metab 42:185–199, 1976

Wetterberg L, Aperia B, Beck-Friis J, et al: Melatonin and cortisol levels in psychiatric illness. Lancet 2:100, 1982

Wetzel RD, Reich T, McClure JN, et al: Premenstrual affective syndrome and affective disorder. Br J Psychiatry 127:219–221, 1975

Wirz-Justice A, Arendt J: Diurnal, menstrual cycle and seasonal indole rhythms in man and their modification in affective disorders, in Biological Psychiatry Today. Edited by Obiols J, Ballús C, Gonzàles Monclús E, et al. Amsterdam, Elsevier North-Holland, 1979, pp 294–302

Chapter 8

Melatonin Rhythm Disturbances in Mood Disorders and Sleep

Steven P. James, M.D.

Chapter 8

Melatonin Rhythm Disturbances in Mood Disorders and Sleep

We live in a physical environment that is continuously changing. The daily rotation of the earth around its axis, the monthly movement of the moon around the earth, and the yearly travel of the earth around the sun are major geophysical changes that constantly influence living organisms. These periodic geophysical changes affect even the smallest units of life. The responses of living organisms to these changes are referred to as biological rhythms.

We can only speculate about the evolutionary reason for the development of biological rhythms, but the ability to anticipate changes in the environment (e.g., day night or summer winter) would have obvious advantages for organisms competing for survival. Thus, rhythmic changes in biological functions may serve to predict environmental changes. To anticipate future conditions, such rhythms must be self-sustaining and driven by an internal clock. Biological rhythms thus represent the hands of an endogenous clock or oscillator situated within the central nervous system.

SEASONAL AFFECTIVE DISORDER

The observation that light alters depression has led to extensive investigation of the retinal–suprachiasmatic nucleus (SCN)–pineal pathway. There is now considerable evidence that the processing of light through this pathway is altered in affective or mood disorders. The earliest recognition of the influence of light is derived from reports of seasonal variation in depression and suicide. Gaedeken (1911) first reported a seasonal pattern of suicide with an inverse relationship between the Northern and Southern Hemispheres. With suicide as a crude indicator of depression, he speculated that changes in environmental light were an important variable in the occurrence of mood disorders. Later studies by Kevan (1980) and Aschoff (1981) show a peak incidence of suicide in the Northern Hemisphere between late spring and early summer. In another study evaluating depression but not suicide, spring was reported to be the most common time for the occurrence of depression (Eastwood and Stiasny 1978). These observations support the hypothesis that an important factor in some mood disorders is the perception and response to environmental light.

Perhaps the most dramatic effect of light in mood disorders is found in seasonal affective disorder (SAD, or winter depression). SAD is a mood disorder characterized by recurrent episodes of depression in the fall and winter and euthymia or hypomania in the spring and summer. Associated symptoms of excessive sleepiness, carbohydrate craving with weight gain, and social withdrawal frequently accompany mood complaints (Rosenthal et al. 1984).

Since the original case report by Lewy et al. (1982) of the successful treatment with a bright (2,500-lux) full-spectrum light, numerous studies have reported an antidepressant response to bright light in these depressed patients (Hellekson et al. 1986; Jacobsen et al. 1987; James et al. 1985; Terman et al. 1987; Wehr et al. 1986, 1987; Wirz-Justice et al. 1986; also see Chapter 6, this volume). Usually a response occurs within 3 days, and relapse after withdrawal occurs within the same time interval. The time of remission suggests that mechanisms separate from those of antidepressant medications (which generally require several weeks for a response) account for the therapeutic effect of bright light. Although the mechanism for this response is not yet known, the observation that bright light suppresses melatonin but dim light does not has suggested that the amount of melatonin secreted by the pineal may be important in SAD.

Rosenthal et al. (1986) investigated the possibility of hypersecretion of melatonin by exposing eight depressed patients with SAD to bright light from 5:30 to 8:30 A.M. and again from 6:00 to 9:00 P.M. for at least 1 week. After the patients had responded with an at least 50% reduction in their Hamilton Rating Scale for Depression (Hamilton 1960) score, they continued on the lights for 2 additional weeks. During the 2-week interval, the patients were randomized in a balanced, double-blind study and were administered either 2 mg of melatonin or a placebo. The objective of the study was to reverse the suppressant effects on melatonin secretion by the bright light for 1 week with exogenous melatonin administration. An analysis of variance comparing postlight, light plus placebo, and light plus melatonin periods showed no interaction between treatment conditions and/or mood. Although bright light is known to suppress the secretion of melatonin and is used to treat depression, melatonin administration did not negate the antidepressant effect of the bright-light treatment. Mechanisms other than the amount of melatonin secreted must thus account for the pathogenesis of SAD.

In a second study, Rosenthal et al. (1988) further evaluated the role of melatonin by administering the β-blocker atenolol. As noted earlier, norepinephrine release results in the stimulation of cyclic AMP (cAMP) (Romero and Axelrod 1974) and synthesis of *N*-acetyltransferase (NAT) with the conversion of serotonin to melatonin. Atenolol blocks the binding of norepinephrine to the pinealocyte and prevents the secretion of melatonin. In this study, 100 mg of atenolol was given to 18 patients with SAD for 1 week, with placebo administration for a 2nd week in a randomized, double-blind procedure. Melatonin suppression was measured by collecting 24-hour urine samples each week and determining the major urinary metabolite of melatonin, 6-hydroxymelatonin. Although 6-hydroxymelatonin was found to be significantly decreased with atenolol administration, no consistent antidepressant effect was found.

Together, these two studies do not support the hypothesis that hypersecretion of melatonin is involved in the pathogenesis of SAD. This is surprising, and somewhat disappointing, because melatonin secretion is known to be an important regulator of seasonal behavior in other species in the animal kingdom.

A related finding of suppression of cortisol after dexamethasone administration was also reported by James et al. (1986a) in patients pretreated with light and before administration of melatonin in the study by Rosenthal et al. (1986). Patients who did not respond had nonsuppression of cortisol with dexamethasone. Although additional studies need to be conducted, the study by James et al. (1986a) and the studies by Rosenthal et al. (1986, 1988) suggest that several of the endocrine rhythms altered in depression appear normal in SAD.

In addition to evaluating the effects of manipulating melatonin secretion in symptomatic SAD patients, we compared the secretory pattern of melatonin in SAD patients and control subjects during the summer and again during the winter. Ten patients previously diagnosed as having SAD and who had a prior response to light in the winter were age- and sex-matched to control subjects. All subjects were exposed for 1 week in the summer to a bright light from 7 to 8 A.M. and again from 8:30 to 9:30 P.M. before hourly samples of melatonin were obtained between 4 P.M. and 9 A.M. The study was repeated again during the winter with light exposure between 7 and 8 A.M. and 4:30 and 5:30 P.M. Blood samples for melatonin determination again were obtained between 4 P.M. and 9 A.M.

No differences in the amplitude of melatonin secretion were found between the summer and winter samplings in SAD patients or in control subjects. Further, no differences between the groups were noted. Because earlier studies had indicated that depressed patients had changes in melatonin secretion when compared with control subjects, the lack of differences (either high or low melatonin) was surprising. Moreover, the absence of changes in melatonin secretory patterns between euthymic periods in the summer and symptomatic episodes in the winter further supports the hypothesis that amount of melatonin secreted during the night is not a causative factor in SAD.

An alternative hypothesis involving melatonin in SAD led to an investigation into the timing of secretion of melatonin (Lewy et al. 1985). This hypothesis, based on a theoretical construct later described by Terman et al. (1987), contained several observations, including the finding that morning light appears superior to light given at other times in reversing the symptoms of SAD. According to this hypothesis, exposure to light in the morning results in a phase advance in the circadian rhythm of melatonin; light in the evening causes a phase delay of the rhythm. Thus, the therapeutic effects of morning light suggest that a phase delay of circadian rhythms in respect to sleep may result in an internal angle disturbance. Exposing patients to morning light may advance the rhythm to a more normal position with the resolution of depressive symptoms in SAD (see Chapter 6, this volume).

To test this hypothesis, Lewy et al. (1985) developed the dim-light melatonin onset method. In this procedure, subjects remain in a dim light in the evening; the onset of the rise in melatonin is determined by frequent blood sampling. With these methods, Lewy et al. (1988) found intriguing changes in SAD patients. These findings suggest that the regulation of the circadian rhythm of melatonin is important in seasonal depression and may have significance in other depressive disorders as well. Until other circadian rhythms (e.g., cortisol and temperature) are examined and their association with the secretion of melatonin determined, the full interpretation of these findings remains unknown (see Chapter 6, this volume). Unfortunately, these additional measurements of circadian rhythm activity have yet to be determined and limit the interpretation of the results.

MELATONIN IN NONSEASONAL DEPRESSION

Numerous observations of alterations in the circadian rhythm of melatonin in patients without SAD suggest that the pineal plays an important role in mood disorders (Beck-Friis et al. 1981; Claustrat et al. 1984; Mendlewicz et al. 1980; Wetterberg et al. 1982; Wirz-

Justice and Arendt 1979). A decrease in the amplitude of the melatonin rhythm at night has been widely reported and seems to occur in both unipolar and bipolar patients (Brown et al. 1985). Wetterberg et al. (1982) have noted that with a decrease of melatonin secretion, an accompanying hypersecretion of cortisol is present. A pineal-hypothalamic interaction is proposed to be involved in the occurrence of depression (see Chapter 3, this volume). However, Branchey et al. (1982) reported that despite the normalization of the cortisol rhythm with the resolution of depressive symptoms, the circadian rhythm of melatonin remains blunted. Thus, the exact interaction between the regulation of the circadian rhythms of cortisol and melatonin remains for future research to clarify.

Although these observations regarding the amplitude of the melatonin rhythm are important, the interpretation of the findings remains limited for several reasons. The early studies were dependent on laboratory methods that, in comparison to current practice, were difficult and unreliable. Daytime values that exceeded nighttime results were frequently found, calling into question the reliability of the assay. Further, with the exception of the 1985 study by Beck-Friis et al., depressed patients were not closely matched by age and sex to control subjects. Nair et al. (1986) and Iguchi et al. (1982) noted that overnight melatonin secretion decreased with increasing age. Thus, the differences reported in depression may have been the result of age differences rather than diagnoses.

Just as age may influence pineal activity, other factors may also affect the secretory pattern of melatonin. Exogenous events including light, sleep, meals, activity, and posture are all known to influence circadian rhythms. As an example, if temperature was being assessed and motor activity was not controlled, any differences found might be the result of behaviors rather than direct influences of a circadian oscillator within the central nervous system. Collectively, these exogenous effects are called masking.

Because light is known to suppress melatonin secretion at night, variation in the exposure to light-dark cycles may mask the rhythm being studied. James et al. (1986b) used a constant routine to evaluate melatonin secretion. Seven depressed patients and seven matched control subjects were placed on strict bed rest for 72 hours. On the first 2 days, all subjects were permitted to sleep between 11 P.M. and 7 A.M., but were sleep deprived for the final 29 hours. Lighting conditions were held constant at 100 lux during waking hours. Diet was controlled by providing patients with hourly feedings calculated to maintain their usual daily calorie intake.

An analysis of the melatonin secretion revealed no differences in either the phase or amplitude of the 24-hour melatonin rhythm in depressed patients or in matched control subjects. When the melatonin rhythm was compared between the first 2 days of normal routine with the 29 hours of constant conditions, no differences between or within groups were found. Although these results differ from the earlier reports that noted changes in melatonin secretion in depression, masking effects do not appear to account for this discrepancy. Thus, unlike other circadian measures such as norepinephrine or temperature, melatonin appears to be a stable endogenous rhythm. Changes in melatonin secretion more likely reflect the activity of a biological oscillator rather than a passive response to environmental influences.

Other investigators also call into question the exact role of melatonin in depression. If the reports of low-amplitude melatonin rhythm are accurate, supplementing the activity of the pineal with exogenous amounts of melatonin could be expected to normalize the rhythm with a resultant change in mood. Although this has not been done after determining blood levels of melatonin, Carmen et al. (1976) did administer exogenous melatonin to depressed patients. Rather than noticing improvement, they found significant deterioration in mood and sleep. Thus, as in SAD, manipulation of blood levels of melatonin by exogenous administration has not resulted in the anticipated findings.

MELATONIN AND SLEEP

Regularity in the timing of sleep and its duration is a rhythmic behavior regulated by complex physiological and psychological factors. The time selected to go to bed and to awaken is clearly influenced by subjective needs, but the tendency to sleep at night and to be active during the day is under a physiological control highly specific to the human species.

The pattern of sleeping at night and being awake in the day is referred to as a diurnal pattern. Other species, including the ground squirrel and the bat, have assumed an ecological niche opposite to our species: they have developed a nocturnal pattern and sleep during daylight. Still others, such as the common house cat, have no demonstrably organized pattern of sleep and are referred to as corpuscular. In addition to timing, the duration of sleep also varies between species. In humans, 6–8 hours of sleep are generally required to be adequately rested. The donkey, however, normally requires only 2 hours of sleep and the opossum 18 hours.

In part because the secretion of melatonin at night occurs at the same time humans need to sleep, the pineal has long been suspected of being involved with sleep. Romijn (1978) commented that the pineal gland may function as a "tranquilizing organ" and serve to turn the central nervous system on and off. This hypothesis had been supported by early investigations of melatonin. Antón-Tay et al. (1971) first gave up to 100 mg of melatonin intravenously to patients with movement disorders. They observed that the patients not only had a reduction in the movement disorders, but also felt sedated. After awakening from their melatonin-induced slumber, mood changes including euphoria were reported. Other studies by Cramer (1980) and Cramer et al. (1974) with 50 mg of intravenous melatonin and Vollrath et al. (1980) with intranasal administration supported these findings. In contrast, Carmen et al. (1976), because of the mood-elevating effects noted by Antón-Tay et al., gave up to 1,200 mg of melatonin orally or intravenously to patients with mood disorders. Rather than seeing an improvement in affect and sleep, they found a deterioration in mood and, on several occasions, psychosis. Although EEG-recorded sleep was not obtained, hourly nursing observation during the night indicated a significant decrease in time asleep.

Despite the differences between these studies, melatonin remains implicated in the regulation of sleep. One major problem in these earlier studies was the unavailability of an assay to determine plasma and cerebrospinal fluid (CSF) levels of melatonin. The development of a sensitive radioimmunoassay by Rollag and Niswender (1976) and the gas chromatography–mass spectrometry method of Lewy and Markey (1978) resulted in the finding that melatonin levels in blood are equivalent to levels in CSF (Reppert et al. 1979) and that oral administration leads to rapid absorption from the gastrointestinal tract.

The availability of sensitive assays to determine endogenous secretion of melatonin (Wetterberg et al. 1978) led to the study by Aldhaus et al. (1985), who evaluated the absorption of melatonin preparations. Both groups found that oral dosages during the day of 1–5 mg of melatonin resulted in plasma levels similar to what naturally occurred during the night. Thus, many of the findings of sleep and mood changes in earlier studies were clearly the result of large pharmacologic effects of melatonin and did not represent the role of melatonin under normal conditions.

James et al. (1987) first reported the effect of a one-time administration of low-dose melatonin at bedtime in 10 normal subjects. In a double-blind, randomized study, either a placebo or a 1-mg or 5-mg preparation of melatonin was given at 1-week intervals 15 minutes before bedtime. Sleep was recorded with standard polysomnographic techniques, and the records were scored with the criteria of Rechtschaffen and Kales (1968). Mood and sleepiness scale ratings were obtained on awakening, and subjects continued to rate their level of sleepiness throughout the day, using the Stanford Sleepiness Scale (Hoddes et al. 1972). Because of the rapid absorption of melatonin and the finding of sedation in earlier studies, the expectation was that the preparations would induce sedation in the subjects. Surprisingly, although placebo administration resulted in a sleep latency of 32.1 minutes and 5 mg of melatonin in a sleep latency of 22.5 minutes, this difference was not statistically significant. Rapid eye movement (REM) sleep latency, however, was found to be 77.2 minutes with placebo and 78.2 minutes with 1 mg of melatonin, but significantly increased to 141 minutes (P < .001) when 5 mg of melatonin was given. Other EEG-determined sleep parameters, including total sleep time, slow-wave sleep, and wakening after sleep onset (WASO) did not show any effect between placebo and either melatonin condition. No changes in mood or level of sleepiness were reported on the subjective scales the following day after the study night. Subjects were also unable to distinguish between placebo and melatonin nights.

A second study with physiologic amounts of melatonin was recently completed by James et al. (in press). In this study, 10 patients with a diagnosis of disorder in initiating and maintaining sleep (without objective findings) were studied (Association of Sleep Disorders Centers 1979). These patients have complaints of insomnia in the presence of little objective differences in sleep. Commonly, the patients subjectively report sleeping 2 or 3 hours, whereas the EEG-determined sleep duration is normal.

With a design similar to our first study on normal subjects, we studied insomniacs with polysomnographic techniques. As in the previous study, sleep latency was 30.3 minutes on placebo, 25.4 minutes on 1 mg of melatonin, and 22 minutes with 5 mg of the compound taken orally. REM sleep latency again was changed with a REM sleep onset occurring 84.5 minutes after sleep onset with placebo, 113.9 minutes after 1 mg of melatonin (P < .05), and 66.7 minutes after 5 mg of melatonin (NS). No change in total sleep time, WASO, or slow-wave sleep was found. In contrast to the study of normal subjects, the insomniacs reported less sleep with increasing dosages of melatonin. Despite this subjective sense of sleep loss, as a group the patients felt that the quality of sleep was better when they were taking melatonin. A review of the mood and behavior scales did not show any change in depression or anxiety among the three conditions that could account for these findings. Thus, it is possible that, rather than changing the duration of sleep, melatonin may alter the perception of being awake or asleep.

The finding of delaying REM sleep onset after nighttime melatonin administration in our two studies is at variance with other studies. Antón-Tay (1974) reported an increase in REM density in humans after large pharmacologic dosages of melatonin. Goldstein and Pavel (1981) found a species-dependent effect in the administration of melatonin, with an increased duration of REM sleep in humans, but a reduction in REM sleep in cats. The significance of these studies is currently unsettled. Dosage, route of administration, species, and acute versus longitudinal administration may account for the differences in REM sleep reported. However, the findings are supportive of the hypothesis that melatonin exerts an important influence on REM sleep and may also be involved in the regulation of other biological rhythms.

CONCLUSION

The secretion of melatonin by the pineal gland is a biological rhythm that represents the activity of the biological clock. As originally described by Lerner et al. (1958), melatonin is synthesized in the pineal from tryptophan. Through 5-hydroxylation and decarboxylation, tryptophan is converted into 5-hydroxytryptamine (serotonin). During the day, the amount of serotonin per gram of tissue in the pineal exceeds that of any other site in the body. Within the pineal, serotonin ultimately has several metabolic fates. The primary one is believed to be conversion into melatonin after N-acetylation by NAT and O-methylation by hydroxyindole-O-methyltransferase (HIOMT) (Wurtman et al. 1963). Presently undetermined in humans, animal studies have indicated that the conversion of serotonin into N-acetylserotonin by NAT is a rate-limiting step (Klein and Moore 1979). At night, the pineal content of NAT increases in tandem with melatonin. During the daylight hours, melatonin and NAT are both dramatically decreased (see Chapter 2, this volume).

The pineal gland is an anatomical structure situated in the epithalamus of the brain. However, the major secretory route of melatonin from the pineal is into the bloodstream. A rich vascular network surrounds the pineal and facilitates its role as a neuroendocrine gland (Ariens Kappers 1960). Although the pineal is a contiguous part of the brain, it extends outside the blood-brain barrier and may directly regulate peripheral function. Examination of CSF samples has found higher concentrations of melatonin in blood than in CSF and supports the belief that secretion of melatonin into the brain from the pineal is not accomplished directly (Arendt et al. 1977; Vaughan et al. 1978). Further work compared cisternal and lumbar spinal fluid and failed to demonstrate a gradient difference, indicating that blood is the major secretory pathway for melatonin (Brown et al. 1979).

The activation of β-adrenergic receptors by norepinephrine is known to initiate a cascade of events in the pineal that lead to the release of melatonin (Brownstein and Axelrod 1974). Stimulation of the β-adrenergic receptors initiates the release of cAMP and induces messenger RNA (mRNA) formation (Romero et al. 1975). With mRNA present, NAT is then increased and the conversion of serotonin to N-acetylserotonin proceeds.

The light-dark cycle influences the release of norepinephrine and the subsequent secretion of melatonin through a complex neurologic network. Although the perception in changes of environmental light can be mediated in lower organisms through nonretinal receptors, in mammals the retina appears critical. Synaptic connections from the cell bodies of the rods and cones to bipolar and horizontal cells occur in the outer plexiform layer of the retina. Associations from the bipolar cells to ganglion cells occur and project into the retinohypothalamic tract (RHT).

Fibers in the RHT are relayed to the SCN, which is situated above the optic chiasm in the anterior hypothalamus. The SCN is reported to be the site of a biological clock that regulates many rhythmic activities (Moore and Klein 1974). From the SCN, connections run to nuclei in the paraventricular hypothalamus. Projections then descend from the paraventricular nucleus through the medial forebrain bundle and terminate on cells in the intermediolateral column of the spinal cord. Fibers from these cell bodies in the intermediolateral column innervate the superior cervical ganglion. The superior cervical ganglion is a major site of sympathetic input to various areas including the pupil via a plexus associated with the internal carotid artery. Two discrete fiber tracts from the superior cervical ganglion referred to as the nervi conarii ascend and eventually innervate the pineal gland through the release of norepinephrine (Ariens Kappers 1960), with the subsequent secretion of melatonin as the end result (see Chapter 1, this volume).

It is important to realize that, although melatonin secretion is influenced by the light-dark cycle, the diurnal rhythm of the pineal is directly controlled by an endogenous clock, probably in the SCN. The elegant work of Ralph et al. (1971) demonstrated the persistence of a melatonin rhythm in rodents and chickens studied in constant darkness. The continued rhythmic secretion of melatonin in the absence of any variation in environmental conditions clearly established the role of an endogenous oscillator in the expression of the circadian rhythm of melatonin. Later work by Klein and Moore

(1979) and Klein et al. (1983) found that the SCN was the oscillator responsible for the regulation of the melatonin rhythm.

Because of the direct control of the pineal by the SCN and the influence of environmental light in the expression of the circadian rhythm of melatonin, Axelrod (1974) first recognized that the pineal functioned as a neurochemical transducer. The circadian rhythm of melatonin may provide information to other physiological systems regarding the status of the external light-dark cycle. Determination of melatonin rhythm may therefore reflect the internal perception of external conditions and provide a means of assessing the temporal organization of the organism.

REFERENCES

Aldhaus M, Franey C, Wright J, et al: Plasma concentrations of melatonin in man following oral absorption of different preparations. Br J Clin Pharmacol 19:517–521, 1985

Antón-Tay F: Melatonin: effects on brain function. Adv Biochem Psychopharmacol 11:315–324, 1974

Antón-Tay F, Diaz L, Fernandez-Guardiola A: On the effect of melatonin upon human brain: its possible therapeutic implications. Life Sci 10:841–850, 1971

Arendt J, Wetterberg L, Heyden T, et al: Radioimmunoassay of melatonin: human serum and cerebrospinal fluid. Horm Res 8:65–75, 1977

Ariens Kappers J: The development, topographical relations and innervation of the epiphysis cerebri in the albino rat. Zeitschrift fur Zellforsch 52:163–215, 1960

Aschoff J: Annual rhythms in man, in Handbook of Behavioral Neurobiology, Vol 4: Biological Rhythms. Edited by Aschoff J. New York, Plenum, 1981, p 475

Association of Sleep Disorders Centers: Diagnostic Classification of Sleep and Arousal Disorders, Vol 2. Roffwary HP, Chairman. 1979, pp 1–138

Axelrod J: The pineal gland: a neurochemical transducer. Science 184:1341–1348, 1974

Beck-Friis J, von Rosen D, Kjellman BF, et al: Serum melatonin in relation to body measures, sex, age, seasonal variation and use of drugs in patients with major depressive disorders and healthy humans. Psychoneuroendocrinology 9:261–277, 1984

Beck-Friis J, Kjellman BK, Aperia B, et al: Serum melatonin in relation to clinical variables in patients with major depressive disorders: a hypothesis of a low melatonin syndrome. Acta Psychiatr Scand 71:319–330, 1985

Branchey L, Weinberg U, Branchey M, et al: Simultaneous study of 24-hour patterns of melatonin and cortisol secretion in depressed patients. Neuropsychobiology 8:225–232, 1982

Brown R, Young SN, Gauthier S, et al: Melatonin in human cerebrospinal fluid in daytime: its origin and variation with age. Life Sci 25:929–936, 1979

Brown R, Kocsis JH, Caroff S, et al: Differences in nocturnal melatonin secretion between melancholic depressed patients and control subjects. Am J Psychiatry 142:811–816, 1985

Brownstein MJ, Axelrod J: Pineal gland: 24-hour rhythm in norepinephrine turnover. Science 184:163–165, 1974

Carmen JS, Post RM, Buswell R, et al: Negative effects of melatonin on depression. Am J Psychiatry 133:1181–1186, 1976

Claustrat B, Chazot G, Brun J, et al: A chronological study of melatonin and cortisol secretion in depressed subjects: plasma melatonin, a biochemical marker in major depression. Biol Psychiatry 19:1215–1228, 1984

Cramer H: Melatonin and sleep, in Sleep. Edited by Popoviciu L, Asgian B, Badui G. Basel, Karger, 1980, pp 204–210

Cramer H, Rudolf J, Consbruch U, et al: On the effect of melatonin on sleep and behavior in man. Adv Biochem Psychopharmacol 11:187–191, 1974

Eastwood MR, Stiasny S: Psychiatric disorder, hospital admission and season. Arch Gen Psychiatry 35:769–771, 1978

Gaedeken P: Uber die Psychophysiologische bedeutung dar Atmospharischen verhaltnisse, inbesondere des Lichts. Z Psychother Med Psychol 3:129–141, 1911

Goldstein R, Pavel S: REM sleep suppression in cats by melatonin. Brain Res Bull 7:723–724, 1981

Hamilton M: A rating scale for depression. J Neurol Neurosurg Psychiatry 23:56–62, 1960

Hellekson CJ, Kline JA, Rosenthal NE: Phototherapy for seasonal affective disorder in Alaska. Am J Psychiatry 143:1035–1037, 1986

Hoddes E, Dement W, Zarcone V: Development and use of the Stanford Sleepiness Scale. Psychophysiology 10:431–436, 1973

Iguchi H, Kato K, Ibayashi H: Age-dependent reduction in serum melatonin concentrations in healthy human subjects. J Clin Endocrinol Metab 55:27–29, 1982

Jacobsen FM, Wehr TA, Skwerer RA, et al: Morning vs. midday phototherapy of seasonal affective disorder. Am J Psychiatry 144:1301–1305, 1987

James SP, Wehr TA, Sack DA, et al: Treatment of seasonal affective disorder with evening light. Br J Psychiatry 147:424–428, 1985

James SP, Wehr TA, Sack DA, et al: The dexamethasone suppression test in seasonal affective disorder. Compr Psychiatry 17:224–227, 1986a

James SP, Sack DA, Rosenthal NE, et al: Circadian melatonin using an unmasking design. New research abstracts presented at the annual meeting of the American Psychiatric Association, Washington, DC, 1986b

James SP, Mendelson WB, Sack DA, et al: The effect of melatonin on normal sleep. Neuropsychopharmacology 1:41–44, 1987

James SP, Sack DA, Rosenthal NE, et al: Melatonin administration and insomnia. Neuropsychopharmacology (in press)

Kevan S: Perspectives on season of suicide: a review. Soc Sci Med 14:369–378, 1980

Klein DC, Moore RY: Pineal N-acetyltransferase and hydroxyindole-O-methyl transferase: control by the retinohypothalamic tract and the suprachiasmatic nucleus. Brain Res 174:245–262, 1979

Klein DC, Smoot R, Weller JL, et al: Lesions of the paraventricular nucleus area of the hypothalamus disrupt the suprachiasmatic spinal cord circuit in the melatonin rhythm generating system. Brain Res Bull 10:647–652, 1983

Lerner AM, Case JD, Takashi J, et al: Isolation of melatonin, the pineal gland factor that lightens melanocytes. Journal of the American Chemical Society 80:2587–2591, 1958

Lewy AJ, Markey SP: Analysis of melatonin in human plasma by gas chromatography negative chemical ionization mass spectrometry. Science 201:741–743, 1978

Lewy AJ, Kern HA, Rosenthal NE, et al: Bright artificial light treatment of a manic-depressive patient with a seasonal mood cycle. Am J Psychiatry 139:1496–1498, 1982

Lewy AJ, Sack RL, Singer CM: Immediate and delayed effects of bright light on human melatonin production: shifting "dawn" and "dusk" shifts the dim light melatonin onset (DLMO). Ann NY Acad Sci 453:253–259, 1985

Lewy AJ, Sack RL, Singer CM, et al: Winter depression and the phase-shift hypothesis for bright light's therapeutic effects: history, theory and experimental evidence. Journal of Biological Rhythms 3:121–134, 1988

Mendlewicz J, Branchey L, Weinberg U, et al: The 24-hour pattern of plasma melatonin in depressed patients before and after treatment. Community Psychopharmacology 4:49–55, 1980

Moore RY, Klein DC: Visual pathways and the central neural control of a circadian rhythm in pineal serotonin N-acetyltransferase. Brain Res 71:17–33, 1974

Nair NPV, Hariharasubramanian N, Pilapil C, et al: Plasma melatonin—an index of brain aging in humans. Biol Psychiatry 21:141–150, 1986

Ralph CL, Hull D, Lynch HJ, et al: A melatonin rhythm persists in rat pineals in darkness. Endocrinology 89:1361–1366, 1971

Rechtschaffen A, Kales A: A Manual of Standardized Terminology, Techniques and Scoring Systems for Sleep Stages of Human Subjects. Los Angeles, CA, Brain Information Service/Brain Research Institute, 1968, pp 1–60

Reppert SM, Perlow MJ, Tamarkin L, et al: A diurnal melatonin rhythm in primate cerebrospinal fluid. Endocrinology 104:295–301, 1979

Rollag MD, Niswender GD: Radioimmunoassay of serum concentration in sleep exposed to different lighting regimens. Endocrinology 98:482–488, 1976

Romero JA, Axelrod J: Pineal β-adrenergic receptor: diurnal variation in sensitivity. Science 184:1091–1092, 1974

Romero JA, Zatz M, Axelrod J: Beta-adrenergic stimulation of pineal N-acetyltransferase: adenosine 3′,5′-cyclic monophosphate stimulates both RNA and protein synthesis. Proc Natl Acad Sci USA 72:2702–2711, 1975

Romijn HJ: The pineal, a tranquilizing organ? Life Sci 23:2257, 1978

Rosenthal NE, Sack DA, Gillin JC, et al: Seasonal affective disorder: a description of syndrome and preliminary findings with light therapy. Arch Gen Psychiatry 41:72–80, 1984

Rosenthal NE, Sack DA, Jacobsen FM, et al: Melatonin in seasonal affective disorder and phototherapy. J Neural Transm [Suppl] 21:257–267, 1986

Rosenthal NE, Jacobsen FM, Sack DA, et al: Atenolol in seasonal affective disorder: a test of the melatonin hypothesis. Am J Psychiatry 145:52–56, 1988

Terman M, Quitkin FM, Stewart JW, et al: The timing of phototherapy:

effects on clinical response and the melatonin cycle. Psychopharmacol Bull 23:354, 1987

Vaughan GM, McDonald SD, Jordan RM, et al: Melatonin concentration in human blood and cerebrospinal fluid: relationship to stress. J Clin Endocrinol Metab 47:220–223, 1978

Vollrath L, Semm P, Gammel G: Sleep induction on intranasal application of melatonin, in Advances in the Biosciences. Edited by Birau N, Schloot W. Proceedings of the International Symposium on Melatonin 29:327–329, 1980

Wehr TA, Jacobsen FM, Sack DA, et al: Phototherapy in seasonal affective disorder: time of day of melatonin is not critical for antidepressant effects. Arch Gen Psychiatry 43:870–875, 1986

Wehr TA, Shwerer RG, Jacobsen FM, et al: Eye versus skin-phototherapy of seasonal affective disorder. Am J Psychiatry 144:753–757, 1987

Wetterberg L, Eriksson O, Friberg Y, et al: A simplified radioimmunoassay for melatonin and its application to biological fluids: preliminary observations on the half-life of plasma melatonin in man. Clin Chim Acta 86:169–177, 1978

Wetterberg L, Aperia B, Beck-Friis J, et al: Melatonin and cortisol levels in psychiatric illness. Lancet 2:100, 1982

Wirz-Justice A, Arendt J: Diurnal, menstrual cycle and seasonal indole rhythms in man and their modification in affective disorders, in Biological Psychiatry Today. Edited by Obiols J, Ballús C, Gonzàlez-Monclús M, et al. Amsterdam, Elsevier North-Holland, 1979, pp 294–302

Wirz-Justice A, Bucheli C, Graw P, et al: Light treatment of a seasonal affective disorder in Switzerland. Acta Psychiatr Scand 74:193–204, 1986

Wurtman RJ, Axelrod J, Phillips LS: Melatonin synthesis in the pineal gland: control by light. Science 142:1071–1073, 1963

Index